FOURTH EDITION

Strategies for Theory
Construction in Nursing

FOURTH EDITION

Strategies for Theory Construction in Nursing

Lorraine Olszewski Walker, RN, EdD, FAAN
Luci B. Johnson Centennial Professor
School of Nursing
The University of Texas at Austin
Austin, Texas

Kay Coalson Avant, RN, PhD, FAAN
Associate Professor
School of Nursing
The University of Texas at Austin
Austin, Texas

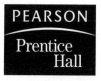

PEARSON

Prentice
Hall

Upper Saddle River, New Jersey 07458

Library of Congress Cataloging-in-Publication Data

Walker, Lorraine Olszewski.
Strategies for theory construction in nursing / Lorraine Olszewski Walker, Kay Coalson
Avant.—4th ed.
p. ; cm.
Includes bibliographical references and index.
ISBN 0-13-119126-8 (pbk.)
1. Nursing—Philosophy. 2. Nursing models. I. Avant, Kay Coalson. II. Title.
[DNLM: 1. Nursing Theory. 2. Models, Nursing. WY 86 W181s 2004]
RT84.5.W34 2004
618.92'85506—dc22
2004049297

Publisher: Julie Levin Alexander
Publisher's Assistant: Regina Bruno
Editor-in-Chief: Maura Connor
Editorial Assistant: Malgorzata Jaros-White
Director of Manufacturing and Production:
Bruce Johnson
Managing Production Editor: Patrick Walsh
Production Liaison: Cathy O'Connell
Production Editor: Trish Finley, Carlisle
Communications
Manufacturing Manager: Ilene Sanford
Manufacturing Buyer: Pat Brown

Design Director: Cheryl Asherman
Cover Designer: Amy Rosen
Senior Design Coordinator: Maria Guglielmo
Walsh
Director of Marketing: Karen Allman
Executive Marketing Manager: Nicole Benson
Channel Marketing Manager: Rachele Strober
Marketing Coordinator: Janet Ryerson
Assistant Editor: Sladjana Repic
Composition: Carlisle Communications

Pearson Education Ltd.
Pearson Education Singapore, Pte. Ltd.
Pearson Education Canada, Ltd.
Pearson Education—Japan

Pearson Education Australia Pty., Limited
Pearson Education North Asia Ltd.
Pearson Educación de Mexico, S.A. de C.V.
Pearson Education Malaysia, Pte. Ltd.
Pearson Education, Upper Saddle River,
New Jersey

10 9 8 7 6 5
ISBN: 0-13-119126-8

This book is dedicated to Charles Bollinger,
who had the courage to say without hesitation,
"Categorically, I like it."
Thanks, Charlie.

Contents

Journal of Child Health Care

http://chc.sagepub.com

Revisiting Goffman's Stigma: the social experience of families with children requiring mechanical ventilation at home

Franco A. Carnevale

J Child Health Care 2007; 11; 7
DOI: 10.1177/1367493507073057

The online version of this article can be found at:
http://chc.sagepub.com/cgi/content/abstract/11/1/7

Published by:
$\bigcirc$ SAGE Publications
http://www.sagepublications.com

On behalf of:

abpn

Association of British Paediatric Nurses

Additional services and information for *Journal of Child Health Care* can be found at:

Email Alerts: http://chc.sagepub.com/cgi/alerts

Subscriptions: http://chc.sagepub.com/subscriptions

Reprints: http://www.sagepub.com/journalsReprints.nav

Permissions: http://www.sagepub.com/journalsPermissions.nav

Citations (this article cites 4 articles hosted on the
SAGE Journals Online and HighWire Press platforms):
http://chc.sagepub.com/cgi/content/refs/11/1/7

Preface

The aim of this book remains the same as at its inception: to provide readers with a resource on theory development written from a nursing point of view. In particular, we have tried to focus on the needs of beginning students of theory development. Stepping into complex philosophic works on the topic can be confusing to those who have had no prior exposure to this subject matter. We have tried instead to provide readers with benchmarks that may be used to start their journey of theory development. The many comments we have received from students support our belief that students benefit from such a resource. We envision this text as a work to be used primarily in nursing graduate programs. Some baccalaureate programs, however, may also find the content of use in integrative senior courses in which students frame their own personal models of practice. As evidenced by citations in the literature, many nurses in addition have found the book useful in developing theory-based programs of research.

In this fourth edition we have tried to strike the balance of retaining substance and adding innovation. Thus, readers will find a number of classics retained in this edition simply because much of the foundational work in theory development was written in an earlier period. To omit such work because of its date of imprint would be intellectually dishonest. At the same time, we have tried to incorporate the burgeoning recent theory development work being done by nurses. Hence, much new material has been added, while many references from prior editions have been relegated to the dustbin.

We have received favorable comments about the introductory pieces at the beginning of each section of the book, so these have been retained and we recommend that readers refer to them for a brief orientation to each of the five sections of the book. We also have added Preliminary Notes at the beginning of each chapter to let us address readers in a more personal voice. This was our need. We hope readers will find this makes the chapters more engaging. Key chapters from the past have been revised and updated.

We have also reordered the chapters focused on strategies into a more intuitive order. Thus, strategies based on synthesis are placed first, followed by derivation, and then analysis. There were two reasons for the reordering. First, we felt that synthesis was actually an easier strategy to learn than analysis. Second, much work has been done with concept and theory analysis over the last few years. We felt that more synthesis and derivation are needed now and in the future to advance the discipline. Furthermore, we hope that the primacy given to the synthesis strategies will encourage development of innovative evidence-based concepts, statements, and theories as a foundation for nursing practice.

In Chapter 13, the final chapter, we have taken a new turn in this edition and focus on what we call frontiers of theory development. This chapter begins with a topic we judged to be of widespread importance: progress in international and ethnicity-related nursing theory. The chapter closes with a look at the tandem areas of nursing informatics and evidence-based practice. We hope that, in particular, our international readers as well as U.S. nurses interested in international aspects of nursing theory will find this chapter of interest. In our search we did not find any similar consideration of international nursing theory development.

In acknowledging those many people who behind the scenes contributed to this edition, we would like to mention the staff of Prentice Hall, specifically Yesenia Kopperman and Sladjana Repic; the staff at Carlisle Communications, including Cindy Miller and Trish Finley; and copy editor Sharon O'Donnell. We also extend our thanks to the following individuals who reviewed this book:

Pattie G. Clark, RN, MSN
Associate Professor of Nursing and Nursing Outreach Coordinator
Abraham Baldwin College
Tifton, Georgia

Susan L. Fickett, RN, MSN
Associate Professor
Saint Joseph's College, Department of Nursing
Windham, Maine

Jean Haspeslagh, DNS, RN
Associate Professor
University of Southern Mississippi
Hattiesburg, Mississippi

Catherine B. Holland, RN, PhD, CNS, ANP, APRN-BC
Associate Professor
Southeastern Louisiana University
Baton Rouge, Louisiana

Elizabeth R. Lenz, PhD
Dean and Professor
The Ohio State University College of Nursing
Columbus, Ohio

Doris Noel Ugarriza, PhD
Associate Professor
University of Miami School of Nursing
Coral Gables, Florida

In our personal network, we owe special thanks to the following: Many thanks to Tim Walker for his steadfast and conscientious help in duplicating, downloading, and printing, as well as sharing Internet access with aplomb. Warm appreciation to Bob and Pauline Medhurst for having room in the inn for this and many other life projects. Many thanks also to Gayle for never-ending patience and encouragement when work on the book interfered with other plans.

L. W.
Austin, Texas

K. A.
Waco, Texas

PART I

Overview of Theory Development in Nursing

In Part I, two chapters present background material to orient readers to the history and language of theory development in nursing. Chapter 1 provides a brief overview of major accomplishments in the field of nursing theory. Four levels of nursing theory development (metatheory, grand theory, middle-range theory, and practice theory) are proposed. Progress that has been made in each level is summarized. The logical distinction between the context of discovery and the context of justification is introduced and related to the need to develop strategies specific to the process of theory generation in nursing. Readers wishing to read primary source materials that have figured in the recent history of nursing metatheory development will find many of these in Reed, Shearer, and Nicoll's (2004) book of readings. Reviews and summaries of substantive theories (or conceptual models) that have been important conceptual landmarks in nursing thought may be found in Fawcett (1993, 1995, 2000), Riehl and Roy (1980), and Fitzpatrick and Whall (1996) among others.

In Chapter 2 the basic vocabulary used in this book is presented and defined. The elements of theorizing (concepts, statements, and theories) are examined in terms of their definitions and relationships to each other and ultimately nursing science. The basic approaches to theory construction (synthesis, derivation, and analysis) are also introduced in Chapter 2. Combining the three elements of theorizing with the three approaches results in nine distinct strategies for theory development: concept synthesis, concept derivation, concept analysis, statement synthesis, statement derivation, statement analysis, theory synthesis, theory derivation, and theory analysis. These form the substance of Parts II, III, and IV of this book. By carefully reading Chapter 2, readers should be able to make a preliminary decision about the strategy or strategies of theory development that are most suited to their needs and interests. Some readers may wish to confine their reading to only the strategies of direct relevance to their work. Others may wish to read all chapters on a given element, such as concepts, or on a particular approach, such as derivation. Last, some readers may simply prefer to read the book from beginning to end out of curiosity (or compulsion). To accommodate these varied reader preferences, we have written the nine strategy chapters so that they are independent of each other except where specifically cross-referenced.

REFERENCES

Fawcett J. *Analysis and Evaluation of Conceptual Models of Nursing.* 3rd ed. Philadelphia, Pa: Davis; 1995.

Fawcett J. *Analysis and Evaluation of Contemporary Nursing Knowledge: Nursing Models and Theories.* Philadelphia, Pa: Davis; 2000.

Fawcett J. *Analysis and Evaluation of Nursing Theories.* Philadelphia, Pa: Davis; 1993.

Fitzpatrick JJ, Whall AL. *Conceptual Models of Nursing: Analysis and Application.* 3rd ed. Stamford, Conn: Appleton & Lange; 1996.

Reed PG, Shearer NB, Nicoll LH, eds. *Perspectives on Nursing Theory.* 4th ed. Philadelphia, Pa: Lippincott; 2004.

Riehl JP, Roy CR, eds. *Conceptual Models for Nursing Practice.* 2nd ed. New York, NY: Appleton-Century-Crofts; 1980.

1

Theory Development in Context

Preliminary Note: *"Why study nursing theory development?" This question has been turned over in the minds of many graduate nursing students. For some, the question is a thoughtful query about new and richer ways of viewing clinical experiences that are deeply familiar. For others, the question forms a challenge for more than superfluous jargon that will be used rarely outside the classroom. For still others, the question conveys an undertone of anxiety about subject matter that looms as daunting and out of reach. In truth, most queries about why the need to study theory development in nursing are an amalgam of all three vantages. Obviously, we cannot satisfy every reader's need for a personalized answer. We attempt in this background chapter, however, to briefly sketch the evolution of nursing theory development to aid readers in formulating their own thoughts and conclusions.*

THEORY DEVELOPMENT AND PRACTICE

Nursing is a practice discipline. Nurses directly engage in providing health care to people at every level of health and illness and at every age. This direct care mission is supported by yet other nurses who educate students, administer educational and service institutions, and develop and test knowledge for practice. The breadth of nursing practice and the varied endeavors that support it show clearly that nursing is a complex discipline. How does theory development relate to the complex and varied dimensions of nursing as a practice discipline?

Simply put, theory development provides a way of identifying and expressing key ideas about the essence of practice. Through theory development that essence may be explored in terms of general or more delimited descriptions and explanations of person, health, environment, and nursing—the metaparadigm concepts that some have argued define nursing as a practice discipline (Fawcett, 1984, 1996). For example, the essence of practice may be studied in a delimited way by focusing on specific events that occur in specific contexts: body image perceptions of adolescent athletes with eating disorders, health promotion behaviors of persons living with HIV, or coping strategies of low-income elders with declining cognitive function. More abstract theory development, by contrast, may focus on the overall architecture of the person–environment relationship as it relates to nursing and health. Regardless of how delimited or grand in scope, theory development is aimed at helping the nurse to understand practice in a more complete and insightful way. Although subsequent chapters in this book provide detailed guidance on the "how" of theory development, beginning students should not lose sight of the "why."

THEORY DEVELOPMENT: A MANDATE FOR EVOLUTION OF NURSING

Early interest in theory development emerged for two reasons. First, nursing leaders saw theory development as a means of clearly establishing nursing as a profession. Theory development was inherent in the long-standing interest in defining nursing's body of knowledge. In a landmark paper early in this century, Flexner defined the characteristics of a profession. Included among Flexner's characteristics were the ideas that professions involve "intellectual operations" and "derive their raw material from science and learning" (quoted in Roberts, 1961, p. 101). Subsequent evaluations of nursing as a profession (Bixler & Bixler, 1945, 1959) specifically examined the extent to which nursing utilized and enlarged a "body of knowledge" for its practice. Indeed, Bixler and Bixler (1945, p. 730) used the term *nursing science* for this knowledge. Interest in the body of knowledge stemmed in part from the extrinsic value of the body of knowledge to nursing as an aspiring profession. As Donaldson and Crowley forcefully stated, "the very survival of the profession may be at risk unless the discipline is defined" (1978, p. 114). However, Dickson (1993) has argued subsequently that "following the male professional model" also has had unintended consequences for nurses. Among these was "reluctance in the workplace to assert and trust nurses' feminine values and views of caring" (p. 80). Nonetheless, developing nursing's distinct knowledge base through theory development, research, and reflective practice was foundational to moving nursing from an occupation subservient to medicine to present-day partnership among the health professions.

Second, interest in theory development was motivated by the intrinsic value of theory for nursing. Simply stated, theory may help nurses grow and enrich their understanding of what practice is and what it can be. The intrinsic value of theory development was reflected in Bixler and Bixler's (1945) first criterion for a profession:

> A profession utilizes in its practice a well-defined and well-organized body of specialized knowledge which is on the intellectual level of . . . higher learning. (p. 730)

Commitment to practice based on sound, reliable knowledge is intrinsic to the idea of a profession and practice discipline. As the integration of professional knowledge, theory provides a more complete picture for practice than factual knowledge alone. Theories that serve as broad frameworks for practice may also articulate the goals of a profession and core values. Consequently, many of the early "grand theories" (see the related section that follows) flowed from attempts to articulate a view of what nursing could be that extended beyond tasks and procedures. Finally, theories that are well developed not only organize existing knowledge but also aid in making new and important innovations to advance practice. For example, Lydia Hall's theoretical work led to many of the nursing practice innovations associated with the Loeb Center for Nursing in New York (Hale & George, 1980).

Systematic reviews of the status of theory development in nursing demonstrate that nursing has made substantial progress in delineating its theoretical base. Fawcett (1983), for example, cited four hallmarks of success in nursing theory development: "a metaparadigm for nursing, conceptual models for nursing, unique nursing theories, and nursing theories shared with other disciplines" (pp. 3–4). In systematically reviewing nursing research articles from 1952 to 1980, Brown, Tanner, and Padrick (1984) noted a trend for authors "to lay explicit claim to a conceptual perspective" (pp. 28–29). Indeed over half the studies they reviewed were judged to contain explicit "conceptual perspectives" (p. 28). Similarly, in a review of nursing research from 1977 to 1986, Moody et al. (1988) found that approximately half of the articles they analyzed contained a "theoretical perspective." Of those, however, non-nursing theories predominated. Several books also have analyzed advances in nursing theory development. Walker (1992) identified and summarized theoretical orientations guiding parent–infant nursing science. In turn, Fawcett (1993) analyzed and evaluated nursing theories that dealt with matters such as deliberative nursing process and human caring. More recently, nursing knowledge that is theory related has been pulled together in Fawcett's comprehensive volume (2000).

Despite the theoretical accomplishments noted above that remain important to the progress of nursing as a practice discipline, much new and continuing work needs to be done. Nurses throughout the world face many questions about nursing and its place in the 21st century. Health care access and financing, need for an adequate workforce of nurses, growth of informatics and technology, and changing health care priorities confront us. An example of theory developed by nurses that is responsive to emerging health care needs is LaCoursiere's (2001) theory of online social support.

Nurses also confront populations of increasingly diverse clients—victims of violence and terrorism, an underclass of poor families struggling to sustain themselves, and a burgeoning population of elders, to mention only a few. These clients come from many different ethnic backgrounds, speak many different languages, and bring new and unexpected health care needs. As members of the largest health profession, nurses have the potential to play leading roles in health care of the future. It is important that they also be clear about nurses' contributions to knowledge development. Thus, although much has been achieved in nursing's theoretical development, the challenge to develop relevant and useful theories to meet the knowledge needs of nurses for the 21st century remains with us.

LEVELS OF THEORY DEVELOPMENT

During the latter half of the 20th century, the desire to develop nursing's theory base launched four levels of theory development literature. The first of these, **metatheory**, focused on philosophical and methodological questions related to the development of a theory base for nursing. The second, **grand nursing theories**, consisted of global conceptual frameworks defining broad perspectives for practice and ways of looking at nursing phenomena based on these perspectives. Third, a less abstract level of theory, **middle-range theory**, emerged to fill the gaps between grand nursing theories and nursing practice. Fourth, a practice-oriented level of theory, **practice theory**, also was advocated. In this fourth level of theory, prescriptions, or, more broadly, modalities for practice were to be delineated. We next sketch out progress made on each of these four fronts. We conclude the summary of the levels of theory development in nursing by proposing a model that depicts how levels of theory development articulate with each other.

Metatheory

Metatheory focuses on broad issues related to theory in nursing and does not generally produce any grand, middle-range, or practice theories. Issues debated at the level of metatheory include but are not limited to (1) analyzing the purpose and kind of theory needed in nursing, (2) proposing and critiquing sources and methods of theory development in nursing, and (3) proposing the criteria most suited for evaluating theory in nursing. Threaded throughout the metatheoretical literature are examinations of the meaning of nursing as a "practice discipline," that is, nursing as both science and profession. An inspection of Table 1–1 shows that metatheory has received extensive attention in nursing. Although some metatheory is accompanied by companion efforts at the grand, middle-range, or practice levels, metatheory has been largely a separate enterprise from these other levels of theory development. Because metatheory represents many points of view about theory in nursing, it has not been consolidated into one unanimously accepted set of beliefs.

Some of the major issues debated in early nursing metatheory were the type of theory suited to nursing, how it should be developed, and the relationship of nursing theory to basic science theories (e.g., Dickoff, James, & Wiedenbach, 1968a, 1968b; Wooldridge, Skipper, & Leonard, 1968). Much of the early understanding of theory development in nursing drew on views of established sciences such as sociology. Recognition of changes in the philosophy of science itself subsequently influenced nursing metatheory. In a critical analysis of the philosophy of science embraced by nursing, Webster, Jacox, and Baldwin (1981) called for "exorcising the ghost of the Received View from nursing" (p. 26). They argued that nurses had uncritically accepted a number of doctrines about the nature of science that were prominent in the 1930s. Based on logical positivism, received view doctrines included beliefs such as "theories are either true or false," "science has nothing to say about values," and "there is a single scientific method" (pp. 29–30). Jacox and Webster (1986) noted the emergence of alternate philosophies of science, including historicism. They suggested that expanding

TABLE 1–1   CHRONOLOGICAL LISTING OF SELECTED METATHEORY IN NURSING

Metatheoretical Paper	Source
Towards Development of Nursing Practice Theory	Wald & Leonard, 1964
The Process of Theory Development in Nursing	McKay, 1965
Symposium: Research—How Will Nursing Define It?	"Research—How Will Nursing Define It?," 1967
Behavioral Science, Social Practice, and the Nursing Profession	Wooldridge et al., 1968
Conference: The Nature of Science and Nursing	"The Nature of Science and Nursing," 1968
Theory in a Practice Discipline	Dickoff et al., 1968a, 1968b
Symposium: Theory Development in Nursing	"Theory Development in Nursing," 1968
Proceedings of the First Nursing Theory Conference	Norris, 1969
Conference: The Nature of Science in Nursing	"The Nature of Science in Nursing," 1969
Proceedings of the Second Nursing Theory Conference	Norris, 1970
Proceedings of the Third Nursing Theory Conference	Norris, 1971
Nursing as a Discipline	Walker, 1971a
Three-Part Series: *Toward a Clearer Understanding of the Concept of Nursing Theory*	Walker, 1971b; Ellis, 1971; Wooldridge, 1971; Folta, 1971; Dickoff & James, 1971; Walker, 1972
Symposium: Approaches to the Study of Nursing Questions and the Development of Nursing Science	"Approaches to the Study of Nursing Questions and the Development of Nursing Science," 1972
Practice Oriented Theory	Advances in Nursing Science, 1978
Critique: *Practice Theory*	Beckstrand, 1978a, 1978b
Theory Development: What, Why, How?	National League for Nursing, 1978
Fundamental Patterns of Knowing in Nursing	Carper, 1978
The Discipline of Nursing	Donaldson & Crawley, 1978
Nursing Theory and the Ghost of the Received View	Webster et al., 1981
The Nature of Theoretical Thinking in Nursing	Kim, 1983
Toward a New View of Science	Tinkle & Beaton, 1983
An Analysis of Changing Trends in Philosophies of Science in Nursing Theory Development and Testing	Silva & Rothbart, 1984
In Defense of Empiricism	Norbeck, 1987
Voices and Paradigms: Perspectives on Critical and Feminist Theory in Nursing	Campbell & Bunting, 1991
The Focus of the Discipline of Nursing	Newman, Sime, & Corcoran-Perry, 1991
(Mis)conceptions and Reconceptions about Traditional Science	Schumacher & Gortner, 1992
Nursing Knowledge and Human Science: Ontological and Epistemological Considerations	Mitchell & Cody, 1992
Postmodernism and Knowledge Development in Nursing	Watson, 1995
A Treatise on Nursing Knowledge Development for the 21st Century: Beyond Postmodernism	Reed, 1995
A Case for the "Middle Ground": Exploring the Tensions of Postmodern Thought in Nursing	Stajduhar, Balneaves, & Thorne, 2001
Nursing Research and the Human Sciences	Malinski, 2002

the philosophical positions adopted in nursing enriched both nursing theories and research.

In a related criticism, Silva and Rothbart (1984) also distinguished between two major schools of philosophy of science, logical empiricism and historicism. They asserted that these two schools differed in several fundamental dimensions, including the underlying conception of science. Logical empiricists, they asserted, emphasize understanding science as a product; historicists understand science from the standpoint of process (pp. 3–5). Similarly, they proposed that logical empiricists and historicists differ in their ideas about the goals of philosophy of science and the components of science. Finally, Silva and Rothbart claimed that logical empiricists assess scientific progress in terms of acceptance or rejection of theories, whereas historicists emphasize the number of scientific problems solved. While noting a stable commitment among nurses to logical empiricism, they acknowledged an emerging diversity in conceptual frameworks and research methods congruent with historicist perspectives.

As nurses reconsidered the metatheoretical assumptions of the discipline, interest in alternate methodologies for nursing theory and research was spawned (e.g., Chinn, 1985; Gorenberg, 1983) to augment more conventional ones. Research methodologists increasingly acknowledged distinct quantitative (Atwood, 1984) and qualitative (Benoliel, 1984) approaches. There are many ways to differentiate these two approaches. One of the most apparent differences is the use of statistical tests in drawing inferences within quantitative approaches and the use of text analysis to portray experiences of participants in qualitative approaches. Some authors proposed integrating both methods within research studies (Goodwin & Goodwin, 1984). The philosophical ferment about the nature and method of science not only was a major focus of nursing metatheory but it also enlarged the approaches advocated for nursing research.

Furthermore, challenges to traditional science by researchers espousing qualitative methods led to clarification of traditional science as understood in nursing. For example, Schumacher and Gortner (1992) corrected common misinterpretations in nursing about traditional science, such as warrants for knowledge claims and universality of laws. Readers who wish more detailed information about philosophy of science and nursing metatheory will find classic reviews in Stevenson and Woods (1986), Suppe and Jacox (1985), and Newman (1992).

Two additional philosophical perspectives introduced into debates about nursing science, theory, and ethics are critical theory and feminism (e.g., Allen, 1985; Campbell & Bunting, 1991; Holter, 1988; Liaschenko, 1993). Both approaches share a common goal of addressing power imbalances inherent in existing social structures that shape the conduct and goals of science as well as human communication.

Critical theory, as applied to nursing (Allen, 1985; Holter, 1988), builds on the philosophic writings of theorists such as Habermas (1971). According to Campbell and Bunting (1991), "In keeping with its Marxist roots, the critical theory epistemology from its inception dictated that knowledge should be used for emancipatory political aims" (p. 4). Critical theory moves beyond existing empirical and interpretive sciences. Through analysis, critical theory reveals ideological positions inherent but unrecognized in existing social structures and scientific methods. For example, qualitative research approaches that stress personal meaning have shortcomings from the perspective of critical theory. "For the critical theorist, personal meanings are shaped by societal structures and communication processes and are therefore all too often ideologic, historically bound, and distorted" (p. 5).

Similarly, feminist approaches aim at realigning social and scientific enterprises in ways that free women from the domination of prevailing, entrenched male structures. As a philosophical approach, feminism is focused at exposing ideology and social conventions that favor men as a group and constrain women as a group. According to Campbell and Bunting (1991), feminist approaches emphasize "unity and relatedness," "contextual orientation," "the subjective," and the "centrality of gender and idealism" (pp. 6–7). Thus, Allen (1985) points out the need to recognize that "one's [scientific] framework is not arbitrary or free of value interests" (p. 64). Finally, Im and Meleis (2001) have explicated six facets of gender-sensitive theories, such as voice and perspective.

Indeed, feminism is part of a broader postmodern philosophical movement challenging modern philosophy and science, including the modern metatheory of nursing. Postmodernism is defined more by rejecting tenets of modern philosophy, than by "any agreement on substantive doctrines or philosophical questions" (Audi, 1995). Because postmodernism undercuts most knowledge derived from traditional scientific methods and rejects "grand narratives," some nursing scholars have called for cautious and thoughtful application of postmodern positions in nursing (Reed, 1995; Stajduhar, Balneaves, & Thorne, 2001). For a historical review of postmodernism and the issues and opportunities it poses for education, practice, and research, see Whall and Hicks (2002).

We believe it is important to carefully consider the philosophical assumptions of present-day nursing theory development and research. We believe it is equally important to put into action principles that form the core of the self-corrective process of science. Central to this core is the idea of the scientific community: scholars who both work in independent research environments yet come together to learn from and examine each other's work. Two principles of operation that have traditionally been used within the scientific community are critique and replication. Thus, scientists actively seek and receive criticism of their work and attempt to reproduce findings independently. These principles serve several purposes, one of which is to maximize the likelihood that human and technical errors in scientific inference will be detected. Philosophical arguments about the received and alternative views of science underscore the need for critique and replication among working scientists. Similarly, philosophical arguments that serve to clarify meaning and purpose need touchpoints with the operational principles guiding the work of nurse scientists. For further readings in the philosophy of science, see the list of additional readings at the close of this chapter.

Grand Nursing Theories

Grand theories are abstract and often have been proposed to give some broad perspective to the goals and structure of nursing practice. Not all grand theories are at the same level of abstraction or have exactly the same scope. On the whole, however, they have as their goal explicating a worldview useful in understanding key concepts and principles within a nursing perspective, yet they are not limited enough to be classified as middle-range theories. In a similar vein, Fawcett (1989) uses the term "conceptual models" for those "global ideas about the individuals, groups, situations, and events of interest to a discipline" (p. 2).

Grand theories have made an important contribution in conceptually sorting out nursing from the practice of medicine by demonstrating the presence of distinct nursing perspectives. Although there may be some disagreement on what works constitute grand theories, Table 1–2 shows a representative listing of writings we would classify as grand theories in nursing.

Most grand theories were developed from the early 1960s through the 1980s. Peplau's (1952) exposition of nursing and its educative function with patients was an early example of grand nursing theory. Grand theories in the 1960s, such as Orlando's *The Dynamic Nurse-Patient Relationship* (1961) and Wiedenbach's *Clinical*

TABLE 1–2   REPRESENTATIVE GRAND NURSING THEORIES

Author(s)	Date	Publication
Peplau	1952	*Interpersonal Relations in Nursing*
Orlando	1961	*The Dynamic Nurse–Patient Relationship*
Wiedenbach	1964	*Clinical Nursing: A Helping Art*
Henderson	1966	*The Nature of Nursing*
Levine	1967	*The Four Conservation Principles of Nursing*
Ujhely	1968	*Determinants of the Nurse–Patient Relationship*
Rogers	1970	*An Introduction to the Theoretical Basis of Nursing*
King	1971	*Toward a Theory of Nursing*
Orem	1971	*Nursing: Concepts of Practice*
Travelbee	1971	*Interpersonal Aspects of Nursing*
Neuman	1974	*The Betty Neuman Health-Care Systems Model*
Roy	1976	*Introduction to Nursing: An Adaptation Model*
Newman	1979	*Toward a Theory of Health*
Johnson	1980	*The Behavioral System Model for Nursing*
Parse	1981	*Man-Living-Health*
Erickson, Tomlin, & Swain	1983	*Modeling and Role Modeling*
Leininger	1985	*Transcultural Care Diversity and Universality*
Watson	1985	*Nursing: Human Science and Human Care*
Roper, Logan, & Tierney	1985	*The Elements of Nursing*
Newman	1986	*Health as Expanding Consciousness*
Boykin & Schoenhofer	1993	*Nursing as Caring*

Nursing: A Helping Art (1964), focused on defining concepts centered in the nurse–patient relationship. For example, Wiedenbach emphasized the patient's "need-for-help" as distinct from nurse-defined patient needs. Orlando differentiated deliberative and automatic nursing actions. These two theorists' work helped nurses clarify and respond to patients' needs and behaviors with the benefit of a theoretical perspective.

Subsequent grand theories shifted from a focus on the nurse–patient relationship to more expansive concepts. For example, Rogers (1970) stressed a holistic perspective on the life process of "man." A multilevel systems model developed by King (1971) included the major concepts of perception, interpersonal relations, social systems, and health. Johnson (1980) constructed a model of the client as a behavioral system composed of seven subsystems. Johnson's thinking was further reflected in Auger's (1976) behavioral systems model, which includes eight subsystems: the affiliative, dependency, ingestive, achievement, aggressive, eliminative, sexual, and restorative. Whereas nurses might deal with medical and physiologic data in the Johnson and Auger grand theories, the approach to these is distinctively a behavioral one.

Later grand theories attempted to capture the phenomenological aspects of nursing. For example, Watson adopted a "phenomenological-existential" orientation in her theory of human care (1985, p. x). Others, such as Leininger's (1985) transcultural care theory, paved the way for nursing's response to more culturally diverse client groups. Development of grand theories also expanded to outside the United States, for example, the Roper-Logan-Tierney theory in the United Kingdom (Roper, Logan, & Tierney, 1985). (See Chapter 13 for other international accomplishments in theory development.)

Although the grand nursing theories provide global perspectives for nursing practice, education, and research, many have limitations. By virtue of their generality and abstractness, many grand nursing theories are untestable in their present form. They may offer general perspectives for practice or curriculum organization in nursing, but by their very nature and purpose most of them would require major revision and expansion before testing would be possible. In revising and refining grand nursing theories, (1) vague terminology would need to be clarified, and (2) interrelationships between concepts in the theories themselves would need to be delineated with sufficient precision so that predictions can be made. Several theorists published revisions of their works in an effort to clarify and further elaborate them (e.g., see King, 1981; Orem, 1995; Roy & Andrews, 1991, 1999; Roy & Roberts, 1981).

Nevertheless, many grand theories pose formidable problems for those wishing to test them. These problems relate to still another problem in grand theories: absent or weak linkages between terminology in the theories and their observational indicators. This is the point on which Suppe and Jacox (1985) critique the tests of the grand theory of Rogers: such tests are contingent on "auxiliary claims that provide most of the testable content" (p. 249). Fawcett and Downs (1986) are even more forceful as they assert that a

conceptual model [and/or grand theory] cannot be tested directly. Rather, the propositions of a conceptual model are tested indirectly through the empirical testing of theories

that are derived or linked with the model. If the findings of theory-testing research sup-
port the theory, then it is likely that the conceptual model is credible. (p. 89)

Thus, it would appear that a layer of theory is needed between grand theories and
their empirical dimensions. This layer is congruent with the idea of middle-range
theory as proposed here. McQuiston and Campbell (1997), for example, have illustrated the process (substruction) whereby an intermediate layer of theory was applied to Orem's (1995) theory to enhance its testability. For detailed analysis and
evaluation of the status (including theory testing) of grand theories such as those of
Johnson, King, Levine, Neuman, Orem, Rogers, and Roy, see Fawcett (1989, 1995,
2000). Also, an extensive review of research guided by the Roy model may be found
in the Boston Based Adaptation Research in Nursing Society (1999).

Although some nurses have focused their work on the problems of testing
grand theories, others have directed their attention to areas of commonality among
grand theories (Flaskerud & Halloran, 1980). Fawcett concluded, "A review of the
literature on theory development in nursing reveals a consensus about the central
concepts of the discipline—person, environment, health, and nursing" (1984,
p. 84). As the broadest area of consensus within the nursing discipline, these concepts constitute its metaparadigm (Fawcett, 1989). In a related vein, Meleis (1985)
identified the following as "domain concepts": nursing client, transitions, interaction, nursing process, environment, nursing therapeutics, and health (p. 184).
Fuller elaboration of some of the metaparadigm concepts was provided by Smith's
(1981) analysis of health's four models, and Kleffel's (1991) exploration of the environmental domain. Others, such as Newman, Sime, and Corcoran-Perry (1991),
however, have put forth alternative versions of the nursing defining foci, with the
concepts of health and caring. Reed (2000), however, critiqued "caring" as overly
focused on nurses' practice and proposed "embodiment" as "a core concept in understanding" patients' experiences of health and illness (p. 131).

Finally, a series of changes in the late 20th century have conspired to put
grand theories somewhat out of vogue. Perhaps because of difficulties in theory
testing (see above), several authors have suggested that a gradual, and perhaps un-
deserved, devaluation of grand theories has occurred in nursing (Barnett, 2002;
DeKeyser & Medoff-Cooper, 2001; Silva, 1999; Tierney, 1998). On another front,
the liberalization of nursing program accreditation criteria pertaining to conceptual frameworks may have contributed to deemphasizing the role of grand theories in nursing education. Finally, growth of postmodern thinking in certain
quarters of nursing has led to the discounting of grand theory as a suitable level of
discourse for nursing. Nevertheless, some nurses have argued that grand theories,
despite their limitations, continue to have merit in the development of the nursing discipline (Barnett, 2002; Reed, 1995; Silva, 1999).

Middle-Range Theories

In view of difficulties inherent in testing grand theories, another more workable
level of theory development has been proposed (Jacox, 1974; See, 1981) and uti-

lized in nursing: theories of the middle range. Theories of this level contain limited numbers of variables and are limited in scope as well. Because of these character-istics, middle-range theories are testable, yet sufficiently general to still be scientif-ically interesting. Thus, middle-range theories share some of the conceptual economy of grand theories but also provide the specificity needed for usefulness in research and practice. Consequently, middle-range theories have gained increasing appeal in nursing research in comparison to grand theories (Lenz, 1998). Although middle-range theories from other disciplines, such as the health belief model (see Champion, 1985; Kviz, Dawkins, & Erum, 1985; Massey, 1986) still are widely used in nursing research (Fawcett, 1999; Lenz, 1998), nursing-based middle-range theories are increasingly evident (Liehr & Smith, 1999). See Table 1–3 for exam-ples of middle-range theories developed in nursing.

Three examples demonstrate the range of middle-range theories developed by nurses. First, Swanson (1991) proposed and refined a theory of caring based on three phenomenological studies. The theory entails five caring processes: know-ing, being with, doing for, enabling, and maintaining belief. Second, Mishel (1988) developed uncertainty theory to explain "how patients cognitively process illness-related stimuli and construct meaning in these events" (p. 225). Uncertainty in-fluences patients' appraisal, coping, and adaptation. Uncertainty itself is influenced by stimuli frame and structure providers. Under certain conditions of continual uncertainty, Mishel (1990) proposes that factors such as social resources aid people to view uncertainty as a "natural" condition. In such a view, "instabil-ity and fluctuation are natural and increase the person's range of possibilities"

TABLE 1–3   EXAMPLES OF MIDDLE-RANGE THEORIES DEVELOPED IN NURSING

Theory	Source
Theory of smoking relapse	Wewers & Lenz, 1987
Uncertainty theory	Mishel, 1988, 1990
Theory of caring	Swanson, 1991
Theory of mastery	Younger, 1991
Theory of culture brokering	Jezewski, 1995
Theory of unpleasant symptoms	Lenz, Suppe, Gift, Pugh, & Milligan, 1995; Lenz, Pugh, Milligan, Gift, & Suppe, 1997
Health promotion model (revised)	Pender, 1996
Theory of nurse-expressed empathy and patient outcomes	Olson & Hanchett, 1997
Theory of chronotherapeutic intervention for pain	Auvil-Novak, 1997
Theory of chronic sorrow	Eakes, Burke, & Hainsworth, 1998
Self-regulation theory	Johnson, 1999
Theory of transitions	Meleis, Sawyer, Im, Messias, & Schumacher, 2000
Theory of comfort	Kolcaba, 2001

(p. 261). Third, Meleis, Sawyer, Im, Messias, and Schumacher (2000) developed a middle-range theory of transitions based on study of ethnically diverse samples undergoing a wide range of transitions. Major categories of variables in the theory include nature of transitions, transitions conditions, and patterns of responses. Transitions conditions include personal factors such as meanings, cultural beliefs and attitudes, socioeconomic status, and preparation and knowledge.

Recently two related, but narrower scope theories, microtheory (Higgins & Moore, 2000) and situation-specific theory (Im & Meleis, 1999), have been introduced into nursing to bring theoretical understanding to delimited clinical situations. Davis and Simms (1992), for example, proposed that microtheory was suitable for procedures involving intravenous therapy and injection administration. Im and Meleis (1999) illustrated the use of situation-specific theory in depicting the experiences of menopause among Korean immigrant women. As these examples show, the focus and range of abstraction of middle-range theories are likely to widen as emerging health needs and advances in science and technology are coupled with increasing diversity of clients served by nurses. (See Hinshaw [2000] for a summary of international nursing research priorities with potential for middle-range theory development.)

Practice Theory

One outgrowth of nursing metatheory has been the idea of a distinct type of theory for nursing as a practice discipline (Dickoff et al., 1968a; Jacox, 1974; Wald & Leonard, 1964; Walker, 1971a, 1971b; Wooldridge et al., 1968). Wald and Leonard (1964) were early proponents of nursing practice theory, a form of theory that was causal in nature and included variables that could be modified by nurses. Jacox (1974), in proposing her idea of practice theory, provided the following succinct description:

> It is theory that says given this nursing goal (producing some desired change or effect in the patient's condition), these are the actions the nurse must take to meet the goal (produce the change). For example, a nursing goal may be to prevent a postoperative patient from becoming hyponatremic. Nursing practice theory states that, to prevent hyponatremia, a particular set of actions must be taken. (p. 10)

The essence of practice theory was a desired goal and prescriptions for action to achieve the goal.

Dickoff and colleagues (1968a) advocated a model of "practice oriented theory" in which four phases of theorizing were to lead to the theory base for nursing practice. These phases included factor-isolating, factor-relating, situation-relating, and situation-producing or prescriptive theory. These four phases roughly paralleled the acts of description, explanation, prediction, and control. Situation-producing or prescriptive theory was comprised of three components: goal content (desired situations), prescriptions, and a survey list. An example of the prescription component offered by Dickoff et al. (1968a) was "Registered nurses, let the patient take his own medication as soon as he is able" (p. 424). The survey list was an intricately developed, yet vague component related to activity.

After the ideas of practice theory, situation-producing theory, or prescriptive theory were proposed, they did not lead immediately to development of any actual theories of this type. Some reasons for the slow growth of these types of theories may be that the early expositions used examples that sounded very procedural and consequently inspired little excitement. Another reason may be that formulating theory for practice requires a well-developed body of nursing science on effective nursing interventions. Consequently, in the intervening years, progress did occur in the knowledge base for nursing practices. For example, in the Conduct and Utilization of Research in Nursing project (Haller, Reynolds, & Horsley, 1979), research-based knowledge was transferred into "protocols for nursing practice" (p. 45). Among the practice protocols studied were (1) sensation information: distress, (2) intravenous cannula change regimen, (3) prevention of decubiti by means of small shifts of body weight, and (4) deliberate nursing: pain reduction. Similarly, clinical guideline statements such as those proposed by the Panel for the Prediction and Prevention of Pressure Ulcers in Adults (1992) provided a further example of statements developed to guide care of persons. Further, several books devoted to nursing interventions have expanded the foundations of nursing practices (Bulechek & McCloskey, 1985; McCloskey & Bulechek, 2000; Snyder, 1992).

Of more recent interest are efforts to blend middle-range theory with prescriptive theory (Good & Moore, 1996). These hybrid efforts elevate the resulting practice theory above simple dictates or imperatives for practice. Although the relational statements of these theories are stated in predictive versus prescriptive (*ought* or *should*) language, they come the closest yet to developing theory that is useful in actual practice. Examples of this emerging version of practice theory are shown in Table 1–4.

Linkages Among Levels of Theory Development

After reading the preceding sections it should be clear that one cannot reasonably ask at what level nursing theory development should occur: Work has been and is being done at each level. A more fitting question is, how are the levels of theory development related to each other? In Figure 1–1 we propose a model of the linkages between and among the four levels of theory development. Metatheory, through analysis of issues about nursing theory, clarifies the methodology and

TABLE 1–4   EXAMPLES OF PRACTICE THEORIES DEVELOPED IN NURSING

Theory	Source
Theory of balance between analgesia and side effects	Good & Moore, 1996
Theory of the peaceful end of life	Ruland & Moore, 1998
Theory of acute pain management in infants and children	Huth & Moore, 1998

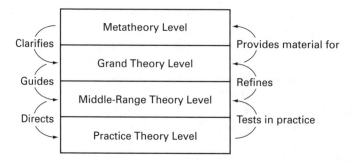

FIGURE 1–1   Linkages among levels of theory development.

roles of each level of theory development in a practice discipline. In turn, each level of theory provides material for further analysis and clarification at the level of metatheory. Grand nursing theories by their global perspectives serve as guides and heuristics for the phenomena of special concern at the middle-range level of theory. For example, Fawcett (1978) used the work of Rogers (1970) to develop a descriptive theory of body image and identification in pregnant couples. Further, middle-range theories, as they are tested in reality, become reference points for further refining grand nursing theories to which they may be connected (see an example of this connection in Gill & Atwood, 1981). Middle-range theories also direct the prescriptions of practice theories aimed at concrete goal attainments. Finally, practice theory, which is constructed from scientifically based propositions about reality, tests (if only indirectly) the empirical validity of those propositions as practices are incorporated in patient care. Those propositions most relevant to practice theory are likely to come from middle-range theories because their language is more easily tied to concrete situations.

Despite the variety of linkages between the levels of theory development, none of them directly represent actual methods or strategies for theory construction. Although metatheory, for instance, illuminates important issues to consider in a developing profession and science, a gap exists between metatheory and methods for actual production of scientific theory. Similarly, the Dickoff et al. (1968a, 1968b) proposal for practice theory does not provide clear and specific procedures to use in constructing a practice theory. Obviously something more is needed to effectively guide nursing toward the construction of its theory base.

THEORY BUILDING: CONTEXT AND METHODS

In this section, we propose two ingredients we believe facilitate the development of nursing theory. These ingredients are focused particularly on producing theory at the middle-range level of generality. We believe that theory development focused at these levels can be facilitated by (1) carefully distinguishing between the context of discovery and the context of justification in constructing theory, and (2) delineating specific strategies and procedures for theory building. These ingredients may not be new in themselves, but we believe that persistent and committed attention to them is.

Contexts of Discovery and Justification

Rudner (1966) used the terms *context of discovery* and *context of justification,* respectively, to differentiate between the processes of developing and evaluating ideas. We, too, believe it is useful to distinguish between the processes of theory construction and theory evaluation. The generation of theory involves initially constructing theory without immediate knowledge of its usefulness or accuracy. Theory evaluation in turn serves to highlight the strengths and weaknesses of a theory by examining the outcomes of theory testing in reality and by comparing the theory with other criteria, such as logical consistency. Prematurely imposing the standards and methods used in theory evaluation upon theory generation can lead to rejection of a promising theory and stifling of the creative process. Further, criticizing the methods or origins from which a theory has been developed because these do not conform to those used in theory evaluation is equally unsound. Although a well-developed theory should be expected to pass review by rigorous standards for theory evaluation, these same standards may not be appropriate for generating theory. For example, small samples or case studies might be employed in developing a theory of early adjustment to parenthood. In testing and evaluating the theory, however, these same data might be judged to be inadequate in size and objectivity. However, disregarding these data during theory generation would be imprudent because valuable insights may be lost. Bearing in mind the difference between development and evaluation frees the theory builder of unnecessary restrictions that might be useful in the context of justification but obstructive in the context of discovery.

Methods of Theory Construction

Clear and explicit methods of theory construction in nursing are needed. Methodologies available in other disciplines, such as sociology (Hage, 1972), have not been translated into a nursing context. In recognition of this need, we have written this methods book. In Chapter 2 our basic framework for strategies of theory development is laid out. In subsequent chapters specific strategies for constructing theory, such as concept synthesis, are described, for the most part, from the vantage point of middle-range theory. The strategies are presented with emphasis on theory construction, not evaluation. Readers interested in theory evaluation are referred to the classic works of Ellis (1968), Hardy (1978), and Barnum (1989).

REFERENCES

Allen DG. Nursing research and social control. *Image.* 1985;17:58-64.
Approaches to the study of nursing questions and the development of nursing science. *Nurs Res.* 1972;21:484-517.

Atwood JR. Advancing nursing science: quantitative approaches. *West J Nurs Res.* 1984;6(3):9-15.

Audi R. *The Cambridge Dictionary of Philosophy.* Cambridge, England: Cambridge University Press; 1995.

Auger JR. *Behavioral Systems and Nursing.* Englewood Cliffs, NJ: Prentice Hall; 1976.

Auvil-Novak SE. A middle-range theory of chronotherapeutic intervention for postsurgical pain. *Nurs Res.* 1997;46:66-71.

Barnett EAM. What is nursing science? *Nurs Sci Q.* 2002;15:51-60.

Barnum B. *Nursing Theory: Analysis, Application, Evaluation.* 3rd ed. Philadelphia, Pa: Lippincott; 1989.

Beckstrand J. The need for a practice theory as indicated by the knowledge used in the conduct of practice. *Res Nurs Health.* 1978a;1:175-179.

Beckstrand J. The notion of a practice theory and the relationship of scientific and ethical knowledge to practice. *Res Nurs Health.* 1978b;1:131-136.

Benoliel JQ. Advancing nursing science: qualitative approaches. *West J Nurs Res.* 1984;6(3):1-8.

Bixler G, Bixler RW. The professional status of nursing. *Amer J Nurs.* 1945;45:730-735.

Bixler G, Bixler RW. The professional status of nursing. *Amer J Nurs.* 1959;59:1142-1147.

Boston Based Adaptation Research in Nursing Society. *Roy Adaptation Model-Based Research: 25 Years of Contributions to Nursing Science.* Indianapolis, Ind: Center Nursing Press; 1999.

Boykin A, Schoenhofer S. *Nursing as Caring: A Model for Transforming Practice;* 1993.

Brown JS, Tanner CA, Padrick KP. Nursing's search for scientific knowledge. *Nurs Res.* 1984;33:26-32.

Bulechek GM, McCloskey JC, eds. *Nursing Interventions: Treatments for Nursing Diagnoses.* Philadelphia, Pa: Saunders; 1985.

Campbell JC, Bunting S. Voices and paradigms: perspectives on critical and feminist theory in nursing. *Adv Nurs Sci.* 1991;13(3):1-15.

Carper BA. Fundamental patterns of knowing in nursing. *Adv Nurs Sci.* 1978;1(1):13-23.

Champion VL. Use of the health belief model in determining frequency of breast self-examination. *Res Nurs Health.* 1985;8:373-379.

Chinn PL. Debunking myths in nursing theory and research. *Image.* 1985;17:45-49.

Davis B, Simms CL. Are we providing safe care? *Canadian Nurse.* 1992;88(1):45-47.

DeKeyser FG, Medoff-Cooper B. A non-theorist perspective on nursing theory: issues of the 1990s. *Scholarly Inquiry Nurs Pract.* 2001;15:329-341.

Dickoff J, James P. Commentary on Walker's "Toward a clearer understanding of the concept of nursing theory": Clarity to what end? *Nurs Res.* 1971;20:499-502.

Dickoff J, James P, Wiedenbach E. Theory in a practice discipline, part I. *Nurs Res.* 1968a;17:415-435.

Dickoff J, James P, Wiedenbach E. Theory in a practice discipline, part II. *Nurs Res.* 1968b;17:545-554.

Dickson GL. The unintended consequences of a male professional ideology for the development of nursing education. *Adv Nurs Sci.* 1993;15(3):67-83.

Donaldson SK, Crowley DM. The discipline of nursing. *Nurs Outlook.* 1978;26:113-120.

Eakes G, Burke ML, Hainsworth MA. Middle-range theory of chronic sorrow. *Image.* 1998;30:179-184.

Ellis R. Characteristics of significant theories. *Nurs Res.* 1968;17:217-222.

Ellis R. Commentary on Walker's "Toward a clearer understanding of the concept of nursing theory": Reaction to Walker's article. *Nurs Res.* 1971;20:493-494.

Erickson HC, Tomlin EM, Swain MAP. *Modeling and Role Modeling: A Theory and Paradigm of Nursing.* Englewood Cliffs, NJ: Prentice Hall; 1983.

Fawcett J. *Analysis and Evaluation of Conceptual Models of Nursing.* 2nd ed. Philadelphia, Pa: Davis; 1989.

Fawcett J. *Analysis and Evaluation of Conceptual Models of Nursing.* 3rd ed. Philadelphia, Pa: Davis; 1995.

Fawcett J. *Analysis and Evaluation of Contemporary Nursing Knowledge: Nursing Models and Theories.* Philadelphia, Pa: Davis; 2000.

Fawcett J. *Analysis and Evaluation of Nursing Theories.* Philadelphia, Pa: Davis; 1993.

Fawcett J. Hallmarks of success in nursing theory development. In: Chinn PL, ed. *Advances in Nursing Theory Development.* Rockville, Md: Aspen; 1983.

Fawcett J. On the requirements for a metaparadigm: an invitation to dialogue. *Nurs Sci Q.* 1996;9:94-97.

Fawcett J. The metaparadigm of nursing: present status and future refinements. *Image.* 1984;16:84-87.

Fawcett J. The state of nursing science: hallmarks of the 20th and 21st centuries. *Nurs Sci Q.* 1999;12:311-318.

Fawcett J. The "what" of theory development. In: *Theory Development: What, Why, How?* New York, NY: National League for Nursing; 1978.

Fawcett J, Downs F. *The Relationship of Theory and Research.* Norwalk, Conn: Appleton-Century-Crofts; 1986.

Flaskerud JH, Halloran EJ. Areas of agreement in nursing theory development. *Adv Nurs Sci.* 1980;3(1):1-7.

Folta JR. Commentary on Walker's "Toward a clearer understanding of the concept of nursing theory": Obfuscation or clarification: a reaction to Walker's concept of nursing theory. *Nurs Res.* 1971;20:496-499.

Gill BP, Atwood JR. Reciprocy and helicy used to relate mEGF and wound healing. *Nurs Res.* 1981;30:68-72.

Good M, Moore SM. Clinical practice guidelines as a new source of middle-range theory: focus on acute pain. *Nurs Outlook.* 1996;44:74-79.

Goodwin LD, Goodwin WL. Qualitative vs. quantitative research or qualitative and quantitative research? *Nurs Res.* 1984;33:378-380.

Gorenberg B. The research tradition of nursing: an emerging issue. *Nurs Res.* 1983;32:347-349.

Habermas, J. *Knowledge and Human Interests.* Shapiro J, trans. Boston, Mass: Beacon Press; 1971.

Hage J. *Techniques and Problems of Theory Construction in Sociology.* New York, NY: Wiley; 1972.

Hale K, George JB. Lydia Hall. In: George JB, ed. *Nursing Theories: The Base for Professional Nursing Practice.* Englewood Cliffs, NJ: Prentice Hall; 1980.

Haller KB, Reynolds MA, Horsley JA. Developing research-based innovation protocols: process, criteria, and issues. *Res Nurs Health.* 1979;2:45-51.

Hardy ME. Perspectives on nursing theory. *Adv Nurs Sci.* 1978;1(1):37-48.

Henderson V. *The Nature of Nursing.* New York, NY: Macmillan; 1966.

Higgins PA, Moore SM. Levels of theoretical thinking in nursing. *Nurs Outlook.* 2000;48:179-183.

Hinshaw AS. Nursing knowledge for the 21st century: opportunities and challenges. *J Nurs Schol.* 2000;32:117-123.

Holter IM. Critical theory. *Scholarly Inquiry Nurs Pract.* 1988;2:223-232.

Huth MM, Moore SM. Prescriptive theory of acute pain management in infants and children. *J Soc Pediatr Nurses.* 1998;3:23-32.

Im E, Meleis AI. An international imperative for gender-sensitive theories in women's health. *J Nurs Schol.* 2001;33:309-314.

Im E, Meleis AI. Situation-specific theories: philosophical roots, properties, and approach. *Adv Nurs Sci.* 1999;22(2):11-24.

Jacox A. Theory construction in nursing: an overview. *Nurs Res.* 1974;23:4-13.

Jacox AK, Webster G. Competing theories of science. In: Nicoll LH, ed. *Perspectives on Nursing Theory.* Boston, Mass: Little, Brown; 1986.

Jezewski MA. Evolution of a grounded theory: conflict resolution through culture brokering. *Adv Nurs Sci.* 1995;17(3):14-30.

Johnson DE. The behavioral system model for nursing. In: Riehl JP, Roy C, eds. *Conceptual Models for Nursing Practice.* 2nd ed. New York, NY: Appleton-Century-Crofts; 1980.

Johnson JE. Self-regulation theory and coping with physical illness. *Res Nurs Health.* 1999;22:435-448.

Kim HS. *The Nature of Theoretical Thinking in Nursing.* Norwalk, Conn: Appleton-Century-Crofts; 1983.

King I. *A Theory for Nursing: Systems, Concepts, Process.* New York, NY: Wiley; 1981.

King I. *Toward a Theory of Nursing.* New York, NY: Wiley; 1971.

Kleffel D. Rethinking the environment as a domain of nursing knowledge. *Adv Nurs Sci.* 1991;14(1):40-51.

Kolcaba K. Evolution of the mid range theory of comfort for outcomes research. *Nurs Outlook.* 2001;49:86-92.

Kviz FJ, Dawkins CE, Erum NE. Mothers' health beliefs and use of well-baby services among a high-risk population. *Res Nurs Health.* 1985;8:381-387.

LaCoursiere SP. A theory of online social support. *Adv Nurs Sci.* 2001;24(1):60-77.

Leininger MM. Transcultural care diversity and universality. *Nurs Health Care.* 1985;6:209-212.

Lenz ER. Role of middle range theory for nursing research and practice. Part I. Nursing research. *Nurs Leadersh Forum.* 1998;3(1):24-33.

Lenz ER, Pugh LC, Milligan RA, Gift A, Suppe F. The middle-range theory of unpleasant symptoms: an update. *Adv Nurs Sci.* 1997;19(3):14-27.

Lenz ER, Suppe F, Gift AG, Pugh LC, Milligan RA. Collaborative development of middle-range nursing theories: toward a theory of unpleasant symptoms. *Adv Nurs Sci.* 1995;17(3):1-13.

Levine M. The four conservation principles of nursing. *Nurs Forum.* 1967;6(1):45-59.

Liaschenko J. Feminist ethics and cultural ethos. *Adv Nurs Sci.* 1993;15(4):71-81.

Liehr P, Smith MJ. Middle range theory: spinning research and practice to create knowledge for the new millennium. *Adv Nurs Sci.* 1999;21(4):81-91.

Malinski VM. Nursing research and the human sciences. *Nurs Sci Q.* 2002;15:14-20.

Massey V. Perceived susceptibility to breast cancer and practice of breast self-examination. *Nurs Res.* 1986;35:183-185.

McCloskey JC, Bulechek GM. *Nursing Intervention Classification (NIC).* 3rd ed. St. Louis, Mo: Mosby; 2000.

McKay RP. *The Process of Theory Development in Nursing.* [dissertation]. New York, NY: Columbia University; 1965.

McQuiston CM, Campbell JC. Theoretical substruction: a guide for theory testing research. *Nurs Sci Q.* 1997;10:117-123.

Meleis AI. *Theoretical Nursing.* Philadelphia, Pa: Lippincott; 1985.

Meleis AI, Sawyer LM, Im E, Messias DKH, Schumacher K. Experiencing transitions: an emerging middle-range theory. *Adv Nurs Sci.* 2000;23(1):12-28.

Mishel MH. Reconceptualization of the uncertainty in illness theory. *Image.* 1990;22:256-261.

Mishel MH. Uncertainty in illness. *Image.* 1988;20:225-231.

Mitchell GJ, Cody WK. Nursing knowledge and human science: ontological and epistemological considerations. *Nurs Sci Q.* 1992;5:54-61.

Moody LE, Wilson ME, Smyth K, Schwartz R, Tittle M, Van Cott ML. Analysis of a decade of nursing practice research: 1977–1986. *Nurs Res.* 1988;37:374-379.

National League for Nursing. *Theory Development: What, Why, How?* New York, NY: National League for Nursing; 1978.

The nature of science and nursing. *Nurs Res.* 1968;17:484-512.

The nature of science in nursing. *Nurs Res.* 1969;18:388-411.

Neuman B. The Betty Neuman health-care systems model: a total person approach to patient problems. In: Riehl JP, Roy C, eds. *Conceptual Models for Nursing Practice.* New York, NY: Appleton-Century-Crofts; 1974.

Newman MA. *Health as Expanding Consciousness.* St. Louis, Mo: Mosby; 1986.

Newman MA. Prevailing paradigms in nursing. *Nurs Outlook.* 1992;40:10-13, 32.

Newman MA. Toward a theory of health. In: *Theory Development in Nursing.* Philadelphia, Pa: Davis; 1979.

Newman MA, Sime AM, Corcoran-Perry SA. The focus of the discipline of nursing. *Adv Nurs Sci.* 1991;14(1):1-6.

Norbeck JS. In defense of empiricism. *Image.* 1987;19:28-30.

Norris CM, ed. *Proceedings of the First Nursing Theory Conference.* Kansas City: University of Kansas Medical Center, Department of Nursing; 1969.

Norris CM, ed. *Proceedings of the Second Nursing Theory Conference.* Kansas City: University of Kansas Medical Center, Department of Nursing; 1970.

Norris CM, ed. *Proceedings of the Third Nursing Theory Conference.* Kansas City: University of Kansas Medical Center, Department of Nursing; 1971.

Olson J, Hanchett E. Nurse-expressed empathy, patient outcomes, and development of a middle-range theory. *Image.* 1997;29:71-76.

Orem D. *Nursing: Concepts of Practice.* New York, NY: McGraw-Hill; 1971.

Orem D. *Nursing: Concepts of Practice.* 5th ed. St. Louis, Mo: Mosby; 1995.

Orlando IJ. *The Dynamic Nurse-Patient Relationship.* New York, NY: Putnam; 1961.

Panel for the Prediction and Prevention of Pressure Ulcers in Adults. *Pressure Ulcers in Adults: Prediction and Prevention.* Clinical Practice Guideline, No 3. Rockville, Md: Agency for Health Care Policy and Research, PHS, USDHHS; May 1992. AHCPR publication 92-0047.

Parse RR. *Man-Living-Health: A Theory of Nursing.* New York, NY: Wiley; 1981.

Pender, NJ. *Health Promotion in Nursing Practice.* 3rd ed. Stamford, Conn: Appleton & Lange; 1996.

Peplau HE. *Interpersonal Relations in Nursing.* New York, NY: Putnam; 1952.

Practice oriented theory, part I. *Adv Nurs Sci.* 1978;1(1):1-95.

Reed PG. A treatise on nursing knowledge development for the 21st century: beyond postmodernism. *Adv Nurs Sci.* 1995;17(3):70-84.

Reed PG. Nursing reformation: historical reflections and philosophic foundations. *Nurs Sci Q.* 2000;13:129-133.

Research—How will nursing define it? *Nurs Res.* 1967;16:108-129.

Roberts MA. *American Nursing: History and Interpretation.* New York, NY: Macmillan; 1961: 101.

Rogers ME. *An Introduction to the Theoretical Basis of Nursing.* Philadelphia, Pa: Davis; 1970.

Roper N, Logan WW, Tierney AJ. *The Elements of Nursing.* 2nd ed. Edinburgh, Scotland: Churchill Livingstone; 1985.

Roy C. *Introduction to Nursing: An Adaptation Model.* Englewood Cliffs, NJ: Prentice Hall; 1976.

Roy C, Andrews HA. *The Roy Adaptation Model.* 2nd ed. Norwalk, Conn: Appleton & Lange; 1999.

Roy C, Andrews HA. *The Roy Adaptation Model: The Definitive Statement.* Norwalk, Conn: Appleton & Lange; 1991.

Roy C, Roberts SL. *Theory Construction in Nursing: An Adaptation Model.* Englewood Cliffs, NJ: Prentice Hall; 1981.

Rudner R. *Philosophy of Social Science.* Englewood Cliffs, NJ: Prentice Hall; 1966.

Ruland CM, Moore SM. Theory construction based on standards of care: a proposed theory of the peaceful end of life. *Nurs Outlook.* 1998;46:169-175.

Schumacher KL, Gortner SR. (Mis)conceptions and reconceptions about traditional science. *Adv Nurs Sci.* 1992;14(4):1-11.

See EM. *Theories of Middling-Range Generality in the Development of Nursing Theory,* Paper presented at the meeting of the Nursing Theory Think Tank, Denver, 1981.

Silva, MC. The state of nursing science: reconceptualizing for the 21st century. *Nurs Sci Q.* 1999;12:221-226.

Silva MC, Rothbart D. An analysis of changing trends in philosophies of science in nursing theory development and testing. *Adv Nurs Sci.* 1984;6(2):1-13.

Smith JA. The idea of health: a philosophic inquiry. *Adv Nurs Sci.* 1981;3(3):43-50.

Snyder M. *Independent Nursing Interventions.* 2nd ed. New York, NY: Delmar; 1992.

Stajduhar KI, Balneaves L, Thorne SE. A case for the "middle ground": exploring the tensions of postmodern thought in nursing. *Nurs Philos.* 2001;2:72-82.

Stevenson JS, Woods NF. Nursing science and contemporary science: emerging paradigms. In: Sorensen GE, ed. *Setting the Agenda for the Year 2000.* Kansas City, Mo: American Academy of Nursing; 1986.

Suppe F, Jacox AK. Philosophy of science and the development of nursing theory. In: Werley HH, Fitzpatrick JJ, eds. *Annual Review of Nursing Research.* 1985;3:241-267.

Swanson, KM. Empirical development of a middle range theory of caring. *Nurs Res.* 1991;40:161-166.

Theory development in nursing. *Nurs Res.* 1968;17:196-227.

Tierney AJ. Nursing models: extant or extinct? *J Adv Nurs.* 1998;28:377-385.

Tinkle MB, Beaton JL. Toward a new view of science. *Adv Nurs Sci.* 1983;5(3):27-36.

Travelbee J. *Interpersonal Aspects of Nursing.* Philadelphia, Pa: Davis; 1971.

Ujhely G. *Determinants of the Nurse–Patient Relationship.* New York, NY: Springer; 1968.

Wald FS, Leonard RC. Towards development of nursing practice theory. *Nurs Res.* 1964;13:309-313.

Walker LO. *Nursing as a Discipline.* [dissertation]. Bloomington: Indiana University; 1971a.

Walker LO. *Parent–Infant Nursing Science: Paradigms, Phenomena, Methods.* Philadelphia, Pa: Davis; 1992.

Walker LO. Rejoinder to commentary: toward a clearer understanding of the concept of nursing theory. *Nurs Res.* 1972;21:59-62.

Walker LO. Toward a clearer understanding of the concept of nursing theory. *Nurs Res.* 1971b;20:428-435.

Watson J. *Nursing: Human Science and Human Care.* Norwalk, Conn: Appleton-Century-Crofts; 1985.

Watson J. Postmodernism and knowledge development in nursing. *Nurs Sci Q.* 1995;8:60-64.

Webster G, Jacox A, Baldwin B. Nursing theory and the ghost of the received view. In: McCloskey JC, Grace HK, eds. *Current Issues in Nursing.* Boston, Mass: Blackwell; 1981.

Wewers ME, Lenz E. Relapse among ex-smokers: an example of theory derivation. *Adv Nurs Sci.* 1987;9(2):44-53.

Whall AL, Hicks FD. The unrecognized paradigm shift in nursing: implications, problems, and opportunities. *Nurs Outlook.* 2002;50:72-76.

Wiedenbach E. *Clinical Nursing: A Helping Art.* New York, NY: Springer; 1964.

Wooldridge PJ. Commentary on Walker's "Toward a clearer understanding of the concept of nursing theory": Meta-theories of nursing: a commentary on Walker's article. *Nurs Res.* 1971;20:494-495.

Wooldridge P, Skipper JK, Leonard RC. *Behavioral Science, Social Practice, and the Nursing Profession.* Cleveland, Ohio: Case Western Reserve; 1968.

Younger JB. A theory of mastery. *Adv Nurs Sci.* 1991; 14(1):76-89.

ADDITIONAL READINGS

Readers who wish to do additional reading in the philosophy of science may find the sources below, many of which are classics, of interest. Introductory readings are preceded by an asterisk (*).

Aronson JL. *A Realist Philosophy of Science.* London, England: Macmillan; 1984.

*Cook TD, Campbell DT. *Quasi-Experimentation: Design & Analysis Issues for Field Settings.* Boston, Mass: Houghton Mifflin; 1979;1-36.

Feyerabend P. *Against Method: Outline of an Anarchistic Theory of Knowledge.* London, England: Verso; 1975.

Giere RN. *Explaining Science: A Cognitive Approach.* Chicago, Ill: University of Chicago Press; 1988.

Glymour C. *Theory and Evidence.* Princeton, NJ: Princeton University Press; 1980.

Harre R. *Varieties of Realism: A Rationale for the Natural Sciences.* New York, NY: Basil Blackwell; 1986.

*Klee R. *Introduction to the Philosophy of Science: Cutting Nature at Its Seams.* Oxford, England: Oxford University Press; 1997

Komesaroff PA. *Objectivity, Science and Society: Interpreting Nature and Society in the Age of the Crisis of Science.* New York, NY: Routledge & Kegan Paul; 1986.

Kuhn TS. *The Structure of Scientific Revolutions.* 2nd ed. Chicago, Ill: University of Chicago Press; 1970.

Lakatos I, Musgrave A, eds. *Criticism and the Growth of Knowledge.* London, England: Cambridge University Press; 1970.

Lamb D, Easton SM. *Multiple Discovery: The Pattern of Scientific Progress.* Trowbridge, England: Avebury; 1984.

Laudan L. *Progress and Its Problems: Toward a Theory of Scientific Growth.* Berkeley: University of California Press; 1977.

*Phillips DC. *Philosophy, Science, and Social Inquiry.* New York, NY: Pergamon; 1987.

Phillips DC. *The Social Scientist's Bestiary: A Guide to Fabled Threats to, and Defenses of, Naturalistic Social Science.* New York, NY: Pergamon; 1992.

Popper KR. *Conjectures and Refutations: The Growth of Scientific Knowledge.* New York, NY: Harper & Row; 1965.

Psillos S. *Scientific Realism: How Science Tracks Truth.* London, England: Routledge; 1999.

Shanker SG, ed. *Philosophy of Science, Logic and Mathematics in the Twentieth Century. Routledge History of Philosophy, Vol. IX.* London, England: Routledge; 1999.

*Suppe F. Response to "positivism and qualitative nursing research." *Scholarly Inquiry Nurs Pract.* 2001;15:389-397.

2

Introduction to Elements, Approaches, and Strategies of Theory Development

Preliminary Note: *"Why do we need strategies for theory construction?" Students and others ask us this question all the time. Our answer has always been the same. Experienced researchers and theorists probably are not even aware of how they put theory together. But novices have to learn how to do it. Learning some systematic ways of examining ideas and putting relationships together allows them to practice until they find ways that work for them.*

Although hard thinking, careful observation, and clear definitions are the best tools of the potential theory builder, they are not enough for the beginner. Structure is helpful when you are a novice or when you are trying a new way to examine a phenomenon. This chapter gives a brief overview of both the elements of theory and the approaches to theory construction.

INTRODUCTION

Both proponents and opponents of organized approaches to theory construction exist. We, of course, believe that using explicit approaches to theory construction can facilitate development of theory. Others would argue otherwise. Opponents see theory development as a non-rule-governed activity. Successful theorizing is, for them, based on the creativity of the theorist. In this line, Hempel (1966, p. 15) argued that there are no rules for mechanically deriving hypotheses or theories from data. We agree with this assertion.

We do not propose to present a set of ironclad rules for theory construction in this book. What we do propose is a comprehensive set of strategies that can augment the intuitive processes that theorists already use in forming concepts, statements, and theories. We see strategies as guidelines for activities. As guidelines, strategies give theorists their bearings but do not remove the burden of creative work from the theorist.

Even good methods, however, cannot salvage a poor idea. In turn, slavishly following a method that is unsuitable can ruin the best of ideas. Users of this book should try to strike a realistic balance between their intuitive processes and the strategies contained herein. As guidelines, the strategies function as points of reference on a creative journey. They are markers along the way to keep the traveler reasonably on course.

To discuss theory building in a meaningful way, we must have some basic understanding among ourselves about the meanings of certain terms that will be used throughout the following chapters. This chapter is devoted to explaining these basic terms and demonstrating, in a general way, how they are related to each other. It is very important to be sure that agreement on meanings of terms is established at the beginning of our discussion.

Three basic elements of theory building and three basic approaches for working with these elements will occupy our attention in this chapter. The three elements are concepts, statements, and theories. The three approaches are synthesis, derivation, and analysis. We will discuss the basic elements first and the approaches later in this chapter. We will demonstrate the relationship of the elements to the approaches in the strategy selection section of the chapter.

ELEMENTS OF THEORY BUILDING

Concepts

Concepts are the basic building blocks of theory (Hardy, 1974). A **concept** is a mental image of a phenomenon, an idea, or a construct in the mind about a thing or an action. It is *not* the thing or action, only the image of it (Kaplan, 1964). Concept formation begins in infancy, for concepts help us categorize or organize our environmental stimuli. Concepts help us identify how our experiences are similar or equivalent by categorizing all the things that are alike about them. Concept formation is thus a very efficient way of learning.

Concepts have different levels of abstractness (Reynolds, 1971). **Primitive concepts** are those that have a common shared meaning among all individuals in a culture. For instance, a primitive concept like the color "blue" cannot be defined other than by giving examples of "blue" and "not blue." **Concrete concepts** are those that can be defined by primitive concepts, are limited by time and space, and are observable in reality. **Abstract concepts** are also capable of being defined by primitive or concrete concepts, but they are independent of time and space (Reynolds). The concept of "temperature," for instance, is abstract, whereas the concept of "temperature today in Kansas City" is concrete because it is dependent on a specific place and time.

Language is the means by which we express a concept. The language "names" (terms or words) we use to express concepts are useful in communicating our ideas to other people. These names or terms are *not* the concepts themselves, they are only our way of communicating the concepts. Thus, the names or terms may be found to be adequate or inadequate at times when we are attempting to get someone to understand our ideas or are trying to define something completely new. If the name or term we are using to attempt to define our concept is inadequate, we may need to refine or change the name, but the concept itself remains the same.

Some authors and researchers use the terms *concept* and *variable* interchangeably. When concepts are defined operationally, that is, the definitions contain within them the means of measuring the concepts, they can be considered "variables" for the purposes of research. Nevertheless, in the context of discussions about theory development, ideas and their names remain "concepts."

Concepts allow us to classify our experiences in a meaningful way both to ourselves and to others. Classifying experiences is a very useful and efficient ability. The ability to express a relationship between two or more concepts is even more useful and efficient. A statement is the result of expressing such a relationship among concepts.

Statements

In any attempt to build a scientific body of knowledge, a **statement** is an extremely important ingredient. It must be formulated before explanations or predictions can be made. A statement, in the context of theory building, can occur in two forms, relational statements and nonrelational statements. A **relational statement** declares a relationship of some kind between two or more concepts. A **nonrelational statement** may be either an existence statement that asserts the existence of the concept (Reynolds, 1971), or a definition, either theoretical or operational.

Relational statements assert either association (correlation) or causality (Reynolds, 1971). Associational statements are simply those that state which concepts occur together. They may even state the direction of the association between concepts, for example, positive, negative, or none. A positive association implies that as one concept occurs or changes, the other concept occurs or changes in the same direction. For example, a positive association is demonstrated by the statement "Palmar sweating increases as anxiety increases." A negative association implies that as one concept occurs or changes, the other concept occurs or changes in the opposite direction. For example, the statement "As anxiety increases, concentration decreases" is a negative association. The "none" relationship implies that the occurrence of one concept tells us nothing about the occurrence of the other concept.

Causal statements demonstrate a cause-and-effect relationship. The concept that causes the change in the other concept may be referred to in research as the independent variable and the concept that is changed or affected, the dependent variable. An example of a causal statement might be "The application of undiluted bleach ($NaOH$) to a colored cotton cloth will cause the color in the cloth to fade."

Adjuncts to relational statements are nonrelational statements. Nonrelational statements are the way by which the theorist clarifies meanings in the theory. **Existence statements** are usually simple statements of assertion about a concept. They are especially useful when the theorist is dealing with highly abstract material. For instance, the assertion "There is a phenomenon known as maternal attachment" is an existence statement. If little was known about the existence of such a phenomenon, it would be helpful to a reader for the theorist to name his or her concept and claim its existence as a starting place in the theory.

The means by which the theorist introduces the reader to the critical defining attributes of each concept is by using **theoretical definitions**. These definitions are usually abstract and may not be measurable. **Operational definitions** reflect the theoretical definitions, but they must have the measurement specifications included (Hardy, 1974). Theoretical and operational definitions are critical in theory building. Without them there is no way to test and thus validate the theory in the "real world."

Theories

The generally accepted definition of a **theory** is an internally consistent group of relational statements that presents a systematic view about a phenomenon and that is useful for description, explanation, prediction, and prescription or control. Associated with the theory may be a set of definitions that are specific to concepts in the theory. Theory is usually constructed to express a new idea or a new insight into the nature of a phenomenon of interest. A theory, by virtue of its predictive and prescriptive potential, is the primary means of meeting the goals of the nursing profession concerned with a clearly defined body of knowledge (Meleis, 1997). That knowledge is a vital component in the human decision-making process involved in evidence-based clinical care and policy formation. However, just because scientific theories may permit control of certain phenomena through relations posited, it does not follow that those theories provide sufficient grounds for using that knowledge as a means of control. It is human judgments about the goals, obligations, and rights of those with whom and for whom care is planned that are the final bases for nurses' use of theory in practice situations.

Description, explanation, prediction, and prescription or control represent different phases of theory development. The ideal theory would do all these things well and simultaneously. However, there is rarely, if ever, such a thing as an ideal theory in any discipline—one that accomplishes all four functions at the same time. Because science is evolutionary and because the human organism is intrinsically fallible, theories are always changing. At any point in time, theories in a discipline may be found at all stages of development. Some theories are specifically designed as explanations, such as the theory of evolution, without any intention of predictability. Others are designed specifically to yield predictability but do not provide prescription or control. Indeed, there are times when prescription or control might be impossible or unethical. For example, major earthquakes can be predicted but not yet controlled and, one hopes, never prescribed. We ought not to despair at this apparently imperfect world of theory building. Scientific thought grows through a self-correcting process. The submission of one's ideas to the critique and analysis of one's colleagues leads to a phenomenon of revision, validation, and extension of any given theory.

The graphic representation of a theory is called a **model**. As Baltes, Reese, and Nesselroade have noted, a model is "any device used to represent something other than itself" (1977, p. 17). The parts of a model should correspond to, or be isomorphic to, the parts of the theory they represent (Brodbeck, 1968, p. 583). A model may be drawn mathematically, as an equation for instance, or it may be

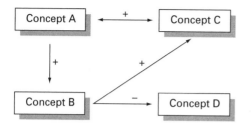

FIGURE 2–1   Schematic model.

drawn schematically using symbols and arrows. A mathematical model might look something like this:

$$Y = {}_{a1}X^{(1)} + {}_{a2}X^{(2)} + {}_{a3}X^{(3)} + E$$

In this equation Y represents a dependent criterion variable, X represents an independent (predictor) variable, each a represents the mathematical weighting applied to the respective X's, and E represents an error term (unexplained variance). A schematic model might look more like Figure 2–1.

Models can be developed either pretheoretically or posttheoretically. The pretheoretical model acts either as a heuristic device or as an attempt by the theorist to discover missing linkages in early theorizing. The posttheoretical model is developed after the theory to lay bare the internal and formal structure of the theory—the system of interrelationships among the concepts.

For the purposes of this book, the term *model* will be used only in its mathematical or schematic sense. This stipulated usage of *model* is necessary to quantify and clarify the relationships between concepts in any theoretical discussions in this book. In some nursing literature, however, *model* may be given a specialized meaning: "the image of the entire field and concepts of all its major units—the goal, patiency, and so forth" (Riehl & Roy, 1980, p 7). In selected nursing literature, the term *model* is reserved for what we have called the "grand theories." For further clarification of levels and types of models, see the Additional Readings at the end of this chapter.

INTERRELATEDNESS OF ELEMENTS

Theory development frequently begins at the level of concepts and statements. For example, in the complete process of theory development, a theorist might start with concept development. As this is accomplished, the goals of statement development and ultimately theory development would be pursued. Only when one has a unified account of a set of relationships, as theories provide, can the goals of prediction and explanation in science be achieved (Hempel, 1966). Theories, of course, need to be tested through research and practice. Testing may in turn highlight

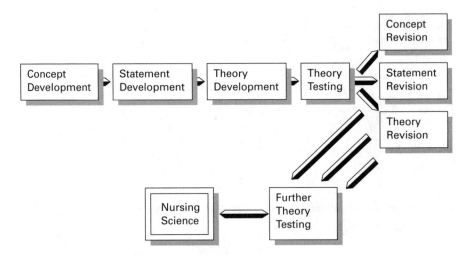

FIGURE 2–2   Phases in the development of nursing science.

areas within theories where revision is needed. At this point the process of theory development is begun again. These phases of theory development are graphically shown in Figure 2–2. Thus, theory development, research, and practice are part of the larger process of the scientific development of a discipline, not separate processes that are ends in themselves. Whereas this book will focus on theory development in nursing, readers should keep in mind the interdependence of theory with research and practice.

APPROACHES TO THEORY BUILDING

Synthesis, derivation, and analysis are the three basic approaches to theory building we use in this book. A theory builder may move back and forth among these approaches; however, we will present them separately to aid the beginner in getting a better picture of each one.

Synthesis

In **synthesis**, information based on observation is used to construct a new concept, a new statement, or a new theory. Synthesis allows the theorist to combine isolated pieces of information that are as yet theoretically unconnected (Bloom, 1956, p. 206). Synthesis works well where a theorist is collecting data or trying to interpret data without an explicit theoretical framework. Much descriptive clinical research consists of collecting large amounts of data in the hope of sifting out important factors and relationships. Synthesis can aid in this sifting process. For example, nurses in school settings might use academic and family information to try to identify factors associated with teenage drug abuse or pregnancy. A researcher might use synthesis to name the clusters in a factor structure or to name the themes in a qualitative data analysis.

Derivation

Analogy or metaphor is the basis of **derivation**. Derivation allows the theorist to transpose and redefine a concept, statement, or theory from one context or field to another. Our strategy of derivation is heavily influenced by the work of Maccia and Maccia (1966) on educational theory models. This approach to theory building can be applied to areas in which no theory base exists. Derivation may also be used in fields in which existing theories have become outmoded and new, innovative perspectives are needed. Derivation provides a means of theory building through shifting the terminology or the structure from one field or context to another. For example, one might take a concept from chemistry, such as chemical equilibrium, and, by analogy, use it to derive a description of how information exchange occurs within a group of professionals.

Analysis

Using **analysis** allows the theorist to dissect a whole into its component parts so they can be better understood (Bloom, 1956, p. 205). In analysis, one clarifies, refines, or sharpens concepts, statements, or theories. Analysis is especially useful in areas in which there is an existing body of theoretical literature. In addition, the theorist examines the relationship of each of the parts to each of the other parts and to the whole. For example, the concept of empathy occurs frequently in the nursing literature. If there are competing or inconsistent points of view about empathy, then an analysis of this concept can help clarify the use, nature, and properties of the concept.

STRATEGY SELECTION

We have superimposed the three approaches to theory building over the three elements of theory. Nine *strategies* for theory building result from this cross-classification of elements and approaches. The strategies and their specific uses in theory building are presented in Table 2–1. By carefully determining the elements of theory desired and the nature of available literature and information on a topic, the theorist may use Table 2–1 as a guide to strategy selection. To determine a suitable theory-building strategy, first of all, the theory builder must be clear about his or her area of interest. Next a theorist must decide whether to focus on concepts, statements, or the overall theory. This will depend on the quality of concept, statement, and theory development that already exists in the area of interest. To determine which *element* best fits their needs, theorists may ask themselves several questions.

1. What is the existing extent of theory development on the topic of interest?
2. How adequate is the existing theory development?
3. In which element is the available theory the weakest: concepts, statements, or the overall theory?

TABLE 2–1 STRATEGIES OF THEORY BUILDING RESULTING FROM CROSS-CLASSIFICATION OF ELEMENTS OF THEORY WITH APPROACHES TO THEORY BUILDING

Elements of Theory	Approaches to Theory Building		
	Synthesis	Derivation	Analysis
Concept	Strategy: Concept synthesis (Chap. 3)	Strategy: Concept derivation (Chap. 4)	Strategy: Concept analysis (Chap. 5)
	Use: To extract or pull together concept(s) from a body of data or set of observations.	Use: To shift and redefine concepts(s) from one field to another.	Use: To clarify or redefine an existing concept.
Statement	Strategy: Statement synthesis (Chap. 6)	Strategy: Statement derivation (Chap. 7)	Strategy: Statement analysis (Chap. 8)
	Use: To extract or pull together one or more statements from a body of data or set of observations.	Use: To shift and reformulate the content or structure of statements from one field to another.	Use: To clarify or refine an existing body of statements.
Theory	Strategy: Theory synthesis (Chap. 9)	Strategy: Theory derivation (Chap. 10)	Strategy: Theory analysis (Chap. 11)
	Use: To pull together a theory from a body of data, set of observations, or set of empirical statements.	Use: To shift and reformulate the content or structure of theories from one field to another.	Use: To clarify or refine an existing theory.

4. What do review articles suggest about the kind of theory development needed next on the topic?
5. What is my personal judgment about the element of theory development that would be the most productive for me to pursue now on my topic of interest?

Carefully consider these questions. Your answers should help you clarify where you should begin theory building: with concepts, statements, or the whole theory.

Selecting the *approach* to be used depends a lot on the extent and type of literature and data available on a topic. Here the theorist may ask another set of questions.

1. Is there any existing literature on the topic?
2. If literature exists, is it research based or purely speculative (untested)?
3. Is the literature tied together by any common conceptual or theoretical frameworks?
4. What do "state of the art" articles suggest about the adequacy of existing theoretical work on the topic? Are new perspectives, organization, or refinement needed?

5. What types of information or data do I have direct access to: clinical observations, field notes, computerized data files?
6. What unique resources do I as theory builder have access to that would facilitate my theory-building efforts: extensive library collection, computer facilities, clinical research projects with ready access to subjects?
7. What is my personal judgment about the approach to theory building that would be the most productive for me to pursue now on my topic of interest?

Carefully examine your answers to these questions. Although more than one approach may be possible, the approach that is the most workable overall should get your first consideration. If the first choice becomes unsatisfactory at a later date, an alternative approach may be considered.

By *putting together* the decision about the *element* of theory and the *approach* most suited to the topic of interest, the choice of a specific *strategy* for theory building should be clear. For example, assume that "empathy" is a topic of interest that showed a need for further work at the concept level. Moreover, assume that analysis appeared best suited for dealing with the extensive literature on this concept (Forsyth, 1979, 1980). Concept analysis would then be a reasonable strategy for further theory building on empathy.

INTERRELATEDNESS OF STRATEGIES

Limiting yourself to only one approach or strategy may not be conducive to successful theory development. As a theory is being constructed, using one strategy may lead you directly to a second strategy that further develops the new theory. We have proposed nine strategies here: concept, statement, and theory synthesis; concept, statement, and theory derivation; and concept, statement, and theory analysis. These nine are not all inclusive of the possible strategies available for use, although they are inherent within most of them (Aldous, 1970; Burr, 1973; Hage, 1972; Zetterberg, 1965). They are our conception of the best strategies to use in nursing theory development in its present state.

No one strategy is going to supply all the needs for theory construction that may arise within one's purview or indeed within the discipline. The theorist will need to determine what the current status of the knowledge base is before selecting a strategy to use. Once the strategy is selected, it should be used until it fails to yield additional information about the topic of interest. When the limits of one strategy are reached, it is time to turn to another strategy. For example, the sequential use of different strategies in the evolution of a theory is exemplified in the development of the theory of unpleasant symptoms (Lenz, Suppe, Gift, Pugh, & Milligan, 1995).

Theory building is iterative. That is, the theorist must continue to use and repeat strategies until the level of desired sophistication in the theory is reached. Hanson (1958) called this iterative process "retroduction." He described the process as using both induction and deduction sequentially to arrive at an adequate theoretical formulation. In effect, Hanson proposed that first the theorist identify several propositions that are fairly specific and induce from them one more general proposition. The second phase of retroduction is to use the new proposition to deduce some new, more specific propositions. This process adds considerably to the body of theoretical knowledge. It is, in fact, the way theory develops in the real world.

We have not attempted to classify these strategies as either inductive or deductive. It seems to us that the only "pure" inductive strategies are the synthesis ones because they are clearly data based. The other strategies, derivation and analysis, may involve theorizing both inductively and deductively. We have preferred to deemphasize the notions of induction and deduction in the strategy chapters, however, in order to keep the strategies as clear and practical as possible. The idea of retroduction makes a great deal more sense to us given the state of the art and the nature of theory in nursing.

Perhaps using some examples here might demonstrate how the strategies can be used interdependently. Let us assume that a theorist reads an article that presents a new theory. A theory analysis helps the theorist understand that the concepts in the theory do not have any operational definitions. The theorist decides to use concept analysis to develop better operational definitions. While using these two analysis strategies, the theorist begins to see possibilities for new relationships among some of the concepts. When he finally decides to formulate statements reflecting those new relationships, the statement synthesis strategy is used.

A second example might be a doctoral student who, during her studies, begins developing a concept she hopes to use in her dissertation. The beginning interest in the concept occurred during the student's clinical practice. After several small field studies, the concept was synthesized. Later, when other concepts needed to be linked to the new one, a statement derivation strategy was used to provide an appropriate structure for the concepts. Finally, after the student graduated, a theory synthesis strategy was ultimately completed. Another theorist, reading the student's discussion of the theory, decided to use it in another discipline, and so theory derivation was used.

A final real-world example is from the Lenz et al. (1995) study mentioned above. Working separately, Pugh and Milligan investigated fatigue in the intrapartum and postpartum periods, respectively. Pugh's study was deductive. Milligan's study was inductive. In discussions, they began to realize that there were many similarities in the two phenomena. They subsequently synthesized the two sets of data plus data from the literature to develop a single framework for studying fatigue in childbearing. In the meantime, Gift and Cahill (Lenz et al., 1995) were studying dyspnea in chronic obstructive pulmonary disease (COPD). Dyspnea and fatigue were found to coexist. Realizing that there was analogic similarity between the concepts of fatigue in childbearing and fatigue in COPD, the investigators analyzed their conceptualizations of fatigue and systematically compared the similarities and differences. Subsequently, after considerable work, they were able to synthesize a theory of unpleasant symptoms from the three data sets, their analyses, and their combined reviews of literature. Thus in the development of the theory of unpleasant symptoms, all three approaches to theory development were used—synthesis, derivation, and analysis.

As you can see from this example, each strategy stands alone and yet each is interdependent with the others. Each strategy provides the theorist with unique information, and yet all of them yield productive ideas for further theory development.

The hallmark of successful theorists is that they allow themselves the freedom to play with ideas or strategies until those ideas or strategies fit the needs of the theorist. As you work with the various strategies, you will become more comfortable with their use. You may even modify some of them or develop new strategies for your theory construction repertoire.

SUMMARY

In this chapter we have dealt with the elements, approaches, and strategies of theory building. The elements of a theory are concepts, statements, and theories. Synthesis, derivation, and analysis are the approaches to theory building. By combining the elements with the approaches, we have constructed a nine-cell matrix of theory-building strategies. Multiple strategies may often be employed before the theory development process is complete.

REFERENCES

Aldous J. Strategies for developing family theory. *J Marriage Fam.* 1970;32:250-257.

Baltes PB, Reese HW, Nesselroade JR. *Life-Span Developmental Psychology: Introduction to Research Methods.* Monterey, Calif: Brooks/Cole; 1977.

Bloom BS, (ed.). *Taxonomy of Educational Objectives. Handbook 1: Cognitive Domain.* New York, NY: McKay; 1956.

Brodbeck M. Models, meaning, and theories. In: Brodbeck, M, ed. *Readings in the Philosophy of the Social Sciences.* New York, NY: Macmillan; 1968:597-600.

Burr JW. *Theory Construction in Sociology of the Family.* New York, NY: Wiley; 1973.

Forsyth GL. Analysis of the concept of empathy: illustration of one approach. *Adv Nurs Sci.* 1980;2(2):33-42.

Forsyth GL. Exploration of empathy in nurse–client interaction. *Adv Nurs Sci.* 1979;1(2): 53-61.

Hage J. *Techniques and Problems of Theory Construction in Sociology.* New York; NY: Wiley; 1972.

Hanson NR. *Patterns of Discovery.* Cambridge, England: Cambridge University Press; 1958.

Hardy ME. Theories: components, development, evaluation. *Nurs Res.* 1974;23:100-107.

Hempel CG. *Philosophy of Natural Science.* Englewood Cliffs, NJ: Prentice Hall; 1966.

Kaplan A. *The Conduct of Inquiry.* San Francisco, Calif: Chandler; 1964.

Lenz ER, Suppe F, Gift AG, Pugh LC, Milligan RA. Collaborative development of middle-range nursing theories: toward a theory of unpleasant symptoms. *Adv Nurs Sci.* 1995; 17(3):1-13.

Maccia ES, Maccia GS. *Development of Educational Theory Derived from Three Educational Theory Models.* Columbus, Ohio: Ohio State University (Project No. 5-0638); 1966.

Meleis AI. Theoretical nursing: definitions and interpretations. In: King I, Fawcett J, eds. *The Language of Nursing Theory and Metatheory.* Indianapolis, Ind: Sigma Theta Tau Honor Society in Nursing; 1997.

Reynolds P. *A Primer in Theory Construction.* Indianapolis, Ind: Bobbs-Merrill; 1971.

Riehl JP, Roy C. Theory and models. In: Riehl JP, Roy C, eds. *Conceptual Models for Nursing Practice.* 2nd ed. New York, NY: Appleton-Century-Crofts; 1980.

Zetterberg HL. *On Theory and Verification in Sociology.* Totowa, NJ: Bedminster Press; 1965.

ADDITIONAL READINGS

Readers who wish to do additional reading about theory and approaches to theory development may find the sources below, many of which are classics, to be of interest. (An asterisk indicates a reference for the advanced reader.)

*Blalock HM. *Theory Construction: From Verbal to Mathematical Formulations.* Englewood Cliffs, NJ: Prentice Hall; 1969.

*Broudy H, Ennis R, Krimerman L, eds. *The Philosophy of Educational Research.* New York; NY: John Wiley; 1973.

Chinn PL, ed. *Advances in Nursing Theory Development.* Rockville, Md: Aspen; 1983.

Chinn PL, Kramer MK. *Theory and Nursing: A Systematic Approach.* 4th ed. St. Louis, Mo: Mosby-Year Book; 1995.

Dubin R. *Theory Building.* 2nd ed. New York, NY: Free Press; 1978.

Fawcett J. A framework for analysis and evaluation of conceptual models of nursing. *Nurs Ed.* 1980;5:10-14.

Fawcett J. The relationship between theory and research: a double helix. *Adv Nurs Sci.* 1978; 1(1):49-62.

Hardy ME. Perspectives on knowledge and role theory. In: Hardy ME, Conway ME, eds. *Role Theory.* New York, NY: Appleton-Century-Crofts; 1978:1-15.

Jacox A. Theory construction in nursing: an overview. *Nurs Res.* 1974;23:4-13.

King I, Fawcett J. *The Language of Theory and Metatheroy.* Indianapolis, Ind: Sigma Theta Tau International Honor Society of Nursing; 1997.

*Kuhn TS. *The Structure of Scientific Revolutions.* 2nd ed. Chicago, Ill: University of Chicago; 1970.

*Lakatos I, Musgrave A, eds. *Criticism and the Growth of Knowledge.* Cambridge, England: Cambridge University Press; 1970.

Meleis AI. *Theoretical Nursing: Development and Progress.* 2nd ed. Philadelphia, Pa: Lippincott; 1991.

Newman M. *Theory Development in Nursing.* Philadelphia, Pa: Davis; 1979.

Newman MA. *Health as Expanding Consciousness.* 2nd ed. New York, NY: National League for Nursing; 1994.

Omery A, Kasper CE, Page GG, eds. *In Search of Nursing Science.* Thousand Oaks, Calif: Sage Publications; 1995

Platt JR. Strong inference. *Science.* 1964;146:347-352.

Rudner R. *Philosophy of Social Science.* Englewood Cliffs, NJ: Prentice Hall; 1966.

Suppe F. *The Semantic Conception of Theories and Scientific Realism.* Urbana: University of Illinois Press; 1989.

Suppe F, Jacox AK. Philosophy of science and the development of nursing theory. In: Werley HH, Fitzpatrick JJ, eds. *Annual Review of Nursing Research.* 3:241–267, New York, NY: Springer; 1985.

Wallace WL. *The Logic of Science in Sociology.* Chicago, Ill: Aldine-Atherton; 1971.

PART II

Concept Development

The very basis of any theory depends on the identification and explication of the concepts to be considered in it. Yet many attempts to describe, explain, or predict phenomena start without a clear understanding of what is to be described, explained, or predicted. Thus sound concept development is a critical task in any effort to develop theory. The next three chapters will focus on ways to develop concepts systematically.

Although we are beginning to see substantial interest in concept development, there is still considerable work to be done in this arena. At least three situations arise in which concept development is needed. The first situation is one in which few concepts or no concepts are available in the theorist's focal area of interest. In this case the theorist must somehow discover, obtain, or invent concepts that are relevant to the phenomenon of concern. Either concept synthesis (Chapter 3) or concept derivation (Chapter 4) would be useful strategies.

When concepts are already available in the area of interest but are unclear, outmoded, or unhelpful, the second situation occurs in which concept development is needed. In this situation the theorist might choose to do a concept analysis (Chapter 5) of one or more of the unclear or unhelpful concepts in an effort to refine and clarify the concept. If the concepts are outmoded, then concept derivation (Chapter 4) might provide new ones that could provide useful insights.

A third situation where concept development might be needed is when substantial theoretical literature or research on a topic exists but are inconsistent. This does not occur often. However, on occasion theorists may be working at one level on an area of interest and researchers or practitioners are working at another level and there is no clear bridge between the two. This has happened in nursing diagnosis work. When it does occur, careful concept development on some of the bridge concepts that link the interests of theorists with practioners and researchers can be very helpful. The most useful strategy for this kind of work is often concept derivation (Chapter 4).

Careful concept development is the basis of any attempt to describe or explain phenomena. It is also prerequisite to any adequate theory. When you are trying to decide where to start with theory development, it might help to ask some questions before you begin. (See the section *Strategy Selection* in Chaper 2.) Discussing issues such as the level of theory development, the type of available literature, and the direction of the literature in the focal area of interest will all provide clues about where to begin. If any of the three situations above are predominant, then one of the concept development strategies is the best place to begin.

The next three chapters describe systematic ways to develop concepts. Each strategy provides a way to understand concepts more thoroughly than you might have done before now. Take your time as you work through these chapters. Allow your mind to be flexible and allow room for playfulness in your thinking. Doing concept work can be fun as well as fruitful.

3

Concept Synthesis

Preliminary Note: *There are increasingly urgent demands for evidence on which to base nursing practice. However, evidence has to be about something. What is that something? The phenomena about which nurses are concerned are the things they deal with on an everyday basis in their work. However, describing, explaining, and predicting about those phenomena has been limited by the inability to name the concepts that represent or capture those phenomena in a way that is easily communicated, or documented. Until we can describe how we think, what we do, and how effective what we do is, we will continue to find ourselves on the defensive related to the evidence about our practice. Concept synthesis is an extremely useful strategy for developing a standard language about our practice.*

DEFINITION AND DESCRIPTION

As in all synthesis strategies, concept synthesis is based on observation or empirical evidence. The data may come from direct observation, quantitative evidence, literature, or some combination of the three. The process of concept synthesis is one of the most exciting ways of beginning theory building. It permits the theorist to use clinical experience as one place to begin.

In a very real sense, you must start from scratch when doing concept synthesis. Concepts are ordered information about the attributes of one or more things that enables us to differentiate among them (Wilson, 1963). Therefore, the theorist using this strategy must invent a new way of grouping, or ordering, information about some event or phenomenon, when the relevant dimensions are unclear or unknown.

Everyone actually does concept synthesis. New concepts often develop from very ordinary activities. Creation of a new concept does not require genius. In fact, all of us who think form new concepts, or categories, as our experiences in the world broaden and increase. When children begin to learn, they begin to place things into categories. These are not always *logical* categories at first, but they become so as the child learns to associate things that are similar in some way. As the child's experience increases, he or she begins to compare new information with the already learned concepts, or categories, of things. If the new information fits one of the previously existing concepts, or categories, it is easily assimilated. If the new information does not fit any previously existing concept or category, then the child must develop a strategy for dealing with the new information. He or she has one of three choices: (1) misname the information by putting it in an old category; (2) deny the new information altogether; or (3) develop a new concept (Breen, 2002; Hunt, 1962; Spitzer, 1977; Stevenson, 1972).

A parent, teacher, or someone else in the child's environment may help in this effort. If a child has always categorized animals with four legs and a tail as "doggie" and then encounters an animal with four legs, a tail, and an udder, goes "moo," and is 4 feet tall, there will be some discrepancy between the new animal and the familiar doggie. The parent may help the child solve the problem by saying "That is a cow." We, as adults, are not always so lucky. When we encounter a new phenomenon in our own experience, there is not always someone around to tell us what the new concept is. We must invent our own name to explain the new phenomenon. This, in effect, is concept formation, the precursor of concept synthesis.

There are several ways to synthesize concepts: (1) by discovering new dimensions of "old" concepts; (2) by examining sets of related concepts for similarities or discrepancies; or (3) by observing new phenomena or clusters of phenomena that have not been described previously. When the discovery of a new concept has been made, a name is chosen or invented that will demonstrate the meaning and allow for pertinent communication about it. The new concept should be defined and its defining attributes delineated so that the reader or user of the new concept can determine what is and what is not intended by the new concept.

PURPOSE AND USES

Concept synthesis is used to generate new ideas. It provides a method of examining data for new insights that can add to theoretical development. New concepts enrich our vocabulary and point to new areas for study.

Historically, Dray's (1959) idea of "explanatory generalizations" is very similar to concept synthesis. He speaks of these explanatory generalizations as occurring in a process of synthesis that "allows us to refer to *x, y,* and *z* collectively as 'a so and so.'" It is, in effect, explaining by finding an appropriate classification for the phenomenon under investigation and naming it. Gordon (1982) has called this same process "pattern recognition." This is a particularly useful strategy for developing nursing diagnoses. In fact, almost any new diagnosis, new syndrome, or new taxonomy represents an attempt at concept synthesis. Whenever a new phenomenon or cluster of phenomena are described empirically or generated from data, the process of concept synthesis has already begun.

Concept synthesis is useful in several areas: (1) in areas where there is little or no concept development; (2) in areas where concept development is present but has had no real impact on theory or practice; and (3) in areas where observations of phenomena are available but not yet classified or named.

APPROACHES TO CONCEPT SYNTHESIS

Qualitative, quantitative, and literary approaches may be used either alone or together to do concept synthesis. Each approach to concept synthesis requires the use of data—qualitative, quantitative, or literary. We will describe each approach and give some relevant examples. Then we will outline the steps of concept synthesis. The steps are the same regardless of the kind of data you use.

Qualitative Synthesis

Qualitative synthesis requires using sensory data such as that gained from listening or observing to obtain information. It speaks to properties of things without assigning a numerical value to the amount of the property present. As the data are collected, they are examined for similarities and differences much as one would in using a grounded theory approach (Benoliel, 1996; Eaves, 2001; Glaser, 1978; Glaser, 1992; Glaser & Strauss, 1967; Kirk & Miller, 1986; Mullen, 1994; Stern, 1994; Strauss & Corbin, 1998). Basically, qualitative synthesis involves recognizing patterns among observations. (For further discussion of qualitative methods see also Chapter 6.)

Denham's (2002) research on family routines is an excellent example of qualitative synthesis. Three ethnographic studies of family routines and rituals were conducted in Appalachia. The first study, of families with preschoolers, yielded seven categories of health routines: dietary practices, sleep and rest patterns, activity patterns, avoidance behaviors, dependent care activities, medical consultations, and health recovery activities. The second study, of families who had lost a family member, yielded five categories: self-care routines, member caregiving, medical consultation, habitual high-risk behaviors, and mental health behaviors. The third study, of disadvantaged families, yielded six categories: self-care routines, dietary practices, mental health, family care, preventive care, and illness care. From these three sets of categories, Denham synthesized six new concepts that described family health routines. The six new concepts were self-care routines, safety and prevention, mental health behaviors, family care, illness care, and member caregiving.

Harris's (1986) study of cultural values and decisions regarding circumcision is another older but still good example of qualitative synthesis. Using a grounded approach, Harris interviewed parents, nurses, and physicians about newborn males. These categories were discovered: circumcision reasoning, cultural decision making, and cultural franchising. These three main concepts were then placed within an explanatory model of cultural decision making about circumcision.

Finally, Kolanowski's study (1995) used qualitative data to extract meaningful clusters of disturbing behaviors manifested by elders with dementia. Five distinct clusters emerged from the study. Kolanowski named the five clusters aggressive psychomotor behavior, nonaggressive psychomotor behavior, verbally aggressive behavior, passive behavior, and functionally impaired behavior.

Quantitative Synthesis

Numerical or statistical data are necessary for **quantitative synthesis.** You may use any studies—experimental or nonexperimental, single case or group designs—as long as they provide quantitative data about the phenomenon of interest. Statistical methods may be employed to extract clusters of attributes comprising a new concept as well as depicting those attributes that do not belong to the concept. Measures such as Q sorts, factor analysis, and Delphi techniques are especially helpful for generating meaningful clusters. Lenz, Suppe, Gift, Pugh, and Milligan's (1995) synthesis of fatigue, reported in Chapter 2, is an excellent example of quantitative synthesis.

Oldaker's 1986 study of normal adolescents' psychological symptomatology is another good example of a quantitative concept synthesis. From several indices of psychological symptoms and personality, Oldaker used principal axis factor analysis to synthesize four concepts related to identity confusion: intimacy, negative identity, diffusion of time perspective, and diffusion of industry.

A classic quantitative study of concept synthesis is that of Kobasa (1979a, 1979b), who studied the effects of life stress on middle- and upper-echelon managers. What she discovered surprised her—of the managers who were identified by high stress levels as at risk for illness, about one third had not had any or at least few illnesses. What made these executives different? Everything Kobasa knew about stress suggested that they should be sick. Was it something in the executives' responses to stressful events that protected them from illness? As a result of these questions, Kobasa set up several studies to collect data on the categories of openness to change, involvement, and control over events. As the data were analyzed the categories were reduced slightly to challenge, commitment, and control. Finally, the concept name "hardiness" was used to accurately reflect the three combined categories. Additional studies have since validated the concept for some occupations but not entirely for others. The studies continue. However, the concept has already made a major impact on stress theory and in nursing (Cataldo, 1993; Kobasa, 1979a, 1979b; Kobasa, Hiker, & Maddi, 1979; Lambert & Lambert, 1987; Nichols & Webster, 1993; Pines, 1980; Wagnild & Young, 1991).

Literary Synthesis

The careful examination of literature is required in **literary synthesis** in order to acquire new insights about phenomena of interest. This examination may yield previously unrecognized concepts for study. Particular to literary concept synthesis is the idea that the literature *itself* becomes the database. Colling's (2000) study of passive behaviors in people with Alzheimer's disease is an example of literary synthesis. Fifteen studies yielded a total of 82 behaviors. The 82 behaviors were then clustered into six initial groupings: diminution of cognition, diminution of psychomotor activity, diminution in feeling emotions, diminution of responding to emotions, diminution of interactions with people, and diminution of interactions with the environment. Next, Colling constructed an instrument using the six categories and with all categories and behaviors defined. She asked a panel of experts in gerontology to sort the behaviors into the categories. The categories were refined and reduced based on results of the analysis of the panel responses. The same six experts then participated in a second round of independent ratings. The final analyses yielded a taxonomy of five independent categories: diminution of cognition, diminution of psychomotor activity, diminution of emotions, diminution of interaction with people, and diminution of interactions with the environment. Finally, the new concepts or categories were evaluated for consistency of use across raters, and for consistency with the Need-Driven Dementia-Compromised Behavior framework (Algase et al., 1996).

A second example is Ryan-Wenger's (1992) study of coping strategies of children. Synthesizing from published studies, Ryan-Wenger developed 15 categories of coping strategies used by children under stress: aggressive activities, behavioral avoidance, behavioral distraction, cognitive avoidance, cognitive distraction, cognitive problem solving, cognitive restructuring, emotional expression, endurance, information seeking, isolating activities, self-controlling activities, social support, spiritual support, and stressor modification (p. 261). Her study is an excellent example of how to verify, or test, a new theoretical formulation.

Mixed Methods

Any of the three approaches to concept synthesis may be used alone or together. There is no hard and fast rule about how or when they may be used. Thus the needs of the theorist and the state of the science are what drive decisions and choices of method. Several recent studies used either single or mixed methods of concept synthesis (Anderson & Oinhausen, 1999; Beitz, 1998; Bunting, Russell, & Gregory, 1998; Colling, 2000; Goldberg, 1998; Kolanowski, 1995; Polk, 1997; Wendler, 1999). The following examples will show how various approaches can be used sequentially or combined to render useful new concepts.

Goldberg (1998) explored the meanings of spirituality using two approaches to concept synthesis. The attributes that arose from the literature on spirituality were meaning, presencing, empathy, compassion, giving hope, love, religion or transcendence, touch, and healing. First, these attributes were clustered into fewer categories. Goldberg then looked at overarching similarities—all implied relationships, either physical or emotional or both. Reviewing the three clusters helped Goldberg realize that a psyche–soma dichotomy was not helpful. The three clusters were thus collapsed into one concept and named "connection."

In a classic study, Clunn (1984) used grounded theory combined with questionnaires to study the cues nurses used to formulate a nursing diagnosis of potential for violence and whether the nurses discriminated between degrees of violent behavior. Using interviews, literature, and scales, 11 concepts were synthesized from Clunn's study: medical history, content of verbalizations, peer relationships, social history, background factors, purposeful motor actions, nonpurposeful motor actions, intensity or emotionality of verbalizations, pervasive affective state, labile emotional reactions, and cognitive indicators of disequilibrium. From these 11 concepts, Clunn synthesized three major factors—interaction, action, and awareness—as the cue categories most used in diagnosing potential for violence. These three factors emerged in both the qualitative and the quantitative portions of the study. Her findings indicated that the actual cues and categories of cues nurses used in assessing the client's potential for violence were similar but the patterns that were salient for some groups of nurses (e.g., emergency room) were not the same as those for other groups (e.g., state hospital).

More recently, Moch (1998), using a series of studies about women diagnosed with breast cancer, her own clinical practice, the literature, and other nurses in practice, synthesized the concept of "health within illness." Moch suggests that health within illness occurs during periods of ill health or compromised well-being. Moch's four attributes for the new concept of health within illness were (1) presents an opportunity, (2) increases meaningfulness, (3) promotes a sense of connectedness or relatedness, and (4) creates awareness of self.

Finally, Burke, Kaufmann, Costello, and Dillon (1991) provided an excellent example of concept synthesis using data from several sources. In their study of the stress of parenting a chronically ill child with repeated hospitalizations, they formed two new concepts. The first was "hazardous secrets," which reflects the parents' perceptions of the parent–health care worker interaction. The parents saw these secrets (e.g., faulty information, gaps in care, and inexperience of the worker) as potentially hazardous to their child. The second concept reflected the process by which the parents managed the stress and was named "reluctantly taking charge" and encompassed vigilance, negotiating rules, calling a halt, and persistent information seeking.

PROCEDURES FOR CONCEPT SYNTHESIS

We will discuss the steps of concept synthesis sequentially but, as in most of the strategies, they are really iterative. That is, you do not always progress from step to step but may cycle through steps several times or go back and forth between steps. Glaser and Strauss (1967) refer to the aim of this process as reaching theoretical saturation. To do this you must become thoroughly familiar with the area of interest by using many resources, including literature reviews and case studies. All provide potential sources of usable data.

During the time you are becoming theoretically saturated, begin to classify the data you acquire. The system of classification need not be rigorous. Indeed, it is better if the system stays fairly loose at this stage. While you are classifying the data, look for clusters of phenomena that seem to relate closely to each other or overlap considerably and combine them. To do this clustering requires only that each classification category be compared to every other category. This can be done using factor analysis on a computer but is not really difficult when done by the theorist using visual inspection.

Once you are satisfied that all the clusters have been discovered and combined where possible, examine the clusters for any hierarchical structure. If there are clusters that appear very similar but one is of a broader nature than the other, it may be helpful to reduce the two clusters into one higher order concept. When the new concept has been reduced as much as possible, a name should be chosen for it that accurately describes it and that facilitates communication about it.

Once the concept is named, the next step is to verify the new concept empirically and modify it as necessary. Verification involves a return to literature, field studies, data collection, and colleagues to discover if the concept is empirically supported. That is, do any of these data sources provide additional information that will expand, clarify, negate, or limit the concept? This process continues until the theorist is satisfied that no new information is being received. At this point the process stops and the new concept is considered adequate. The new concept should then be described in a theoretical definition that includes its defining attributes.

Finally, determine, if possible, where the new concept fits into existing theory in the area. Consideration should be given to the distinctive insights and potential approaches to research and practice the new concept makes possible. There may even be times when a concept is so radically different from current theoretical positions that a whole new field of study emerges. A good example of this effect was the discovery of microbes that generated the field of bacteriology. Sometimes an existing system of thinking is completely changed, as when the concept of relativity completely changed the orientation of the field of physics.

Keeping your working memory updated on current thinking about the phenomena of concern to you is a critical factor that facilitates concept synthesis. It is very important to be thoroughly familiar with one's own field of interest. It is equally important to be able to retain a significant amount of that knowledge in your memory. In this way, phenomena that "don't compute" with existing ways of thinking become more obvious.

However, because memory is fallible, it is very useful for theorists to develop a notebook of memos to themselves. In this notebook, observations should be carefully recorded. These may be directly observed phenomena, statistical findings, or information summaries from literature. Both at the time of writing the memo and at the time the theorist reviews the notebook, insights and interpretations of the data should be added to the memo. These interpretive notes form the basis for developing classifications in initial concept synthesis efforts and in efforts to develop higher concepts at a later time (Schatzman & Strauss, 1973).

The ability to observe is another critical factor that facilitates concept synthesis. Obviously, a keen observer is more likely to see new phenomena than one who never looks. This skill is not inborn. It is acquired with practice. (If you feel you are not a careful observer, try Practice Exercise 1 at the end of this chapter.)

The skill of evaluating evidence is a corollary to the skill of observation. This ability to look at data, determine its value, and extract the new ideas can be learned also. Refer to the additional readings on evaluating research at the end of this chapter or any good research text for honing such perceptions.

Openness to new ideas is the last critical factor that influences concept synthesis. This implies, at least, a freedom from the fear of discovering something new. Many nurses practice nursing precisely as they were taught and have little inclination to question or experiment with new ways of doing or thinking about things. Change to many people is very threatening and certainly synthesizing a new concept will initiate some change, if only in thinking. Therefore, before concept synthesis can occur, the nurse must be willing to allow the possibility of new ideas.

New ideas come to us from all our senses. Most of us are verbally and mathematically trained but have little practice relying on taste, smell, vision, or touch to help us arrive at new ideas. It is often helpful to think divergently by forcing ourselves to use other than our verbal or mathematics skills to arrive at new ideas about phenomena.

Coupled with the idea of using all our senses to help us generate new concepts is the admonition to take plenty of time. The process of synthesis is creating something new; it cannot be accomplished quickly. Ideas take time to develop or "incubate." Relax and don't push yourself.

ADVANTAGES AND LIMITATIONS

Concept synthesis provides a mechanism for creating something new from data already available. It provides new insights and adds texture and richness to the fabric of developing theory. Given the growing interest in electronic patient records and nursing informatics, the naming of nursing phenomena and nursing activities makes concept synthesis especially pertinent. The process of concept synthesis is especially useful as a means of generating and naming potential nursing diagnoses, interventions, and outcomes.

Concept synthesis does take time and requires the theorist to be open to risk taking. The theorist must begin with raw data and attempt to conceive a new idea from it. Sometimes this happens quickly. More often, it happens only after considerable time and thought.

Verifying concepts also takes time. This is when the theorist feels most uncomfortable. What if the new concept can't be verified? The fear of being wrong is powerful, especially when the theorist may view the new concept as a "brain child" and is very attached to it. The necessity here is for the theorist to remain objective and scientific. If the concept is truly data based, it should come through the verification with only minor revisions.

Finally, concepts in themselves are only useful to describe a phenomenon. They do not provide for explanation, prediction, or prescription or control. It is only when concepts are connected to each other through relational statements that we have the possibility of a hypothesis or a theory.

UTILIZING THE RESULTS OF CONCEPT SYNTHESIS

Concept synthesis is useful when there is a need to explain something by classifying it, or when we need wholly new concepts or new uses for old ones. But what do you do with a new concept once you've synthesized it?

Several things can and should be done. The first of these is to verify, support, or validate the new concept (see Chapter 12). This is very much like establishing content validity or transferability in research, and the same methods can be used for either task. Once the concept has attained an adequate degree of support, a good theoretical definition containing the defining attributes should be written. When this is accomplished, the new concept should be shared by publishing it.

Knowledge development in the nursing discipline requires valid new concepts. New concepts are useful in both our science and in our practice. In education, the new concept could be used to describe nursing phenomena to students in a meaningful way or to classify patient needs or nursing actions. In practice the new concept may give clinicians fresh insights into patient problems, new nursing diagnoses, and possible new nursing interventions. In research and theory building, the new concept may provide fruitful new hypotheses or induce a change in thinking about some phenomenon of concern that in turn will generate more research.

SUMMARY

Concept synthesis employs pulling together various elements of data into a pattern or relationship not clearly seen before to form a new whole, a new concept. The steps of concept synthesis include becoming thoroughly familiar with an area of interest, loosely classifying the data you have acquired about the area of interest, looking for and combining clusters of classified phenomena that seem to relate closely or overlap, choosing a name for the cluster that accurately represents the phenomenon and that will facilitate communication about it, verifying the new concept empirically, and determining if or where the new concept fits into current theory and practice.

Concept synthesis is a highly creative activity and may add significant new information to a given area of interest. The strategy is limited by the length of time needed for full concept development and by the fact that concepts alone do not provide predictive potential.

PRACTICE EXERCISES

Exercise 1. Observing

Choose an object in your environment, such as a piece of equipment you use frequently or an object you handle every day. Spend 10 minutes observing the object. Make a list of everything you see about it. How long was your list? If you saw only a few things, go back and spend 10 more minutes observing it. Is your list longer? Did you take apart the object and describe each piece separately? If not, why not? Now, go back and look again. Spend 10 minutes listing all possible uses of the item. How long was the list? Did you describe uses for each *part* of the item as well as for the whole? If not, why not? Learning to be a keen observer requires that our stereotypes be disposed of and that we keep an open and creative mind when we really *look* at something familiar.

Exercise 2. Memory

Without looking at one, draw a telephone keypad. Put in the letters and numbers where they belong (Adams, 1979).

Very few people can do this right the first time. The exercise demonstrates how we may *think* we have all the data we need because we use the phone every day after all, but are so familiar with the object we no longer really *see* it. Try this exercise again with an object you use every day at work. First, draw it without looking, then go back and draw it again while you look at it. How did the two differ?

Exercise 3. Concept Clustering

Below are 28 names of concepts. Make at least two concept clusters from the list.

soap	car	volcano	duck
tennis racket	desk	hat	deodorant
dog	vote	fish	bus
toothbrush	disk	grass	mop
policy	elephant	guidelines	orange
frog	avocado	melody	panpipe
umbrella	basket	bucket	turnip

Exercise 4. Concept Synthesis

In order to facilitate your practice of the steps in concept synthesis, we have structured this exercise more than will be the case in reality. In fact, what we have done here is to present a kind of matrix used in morphologic analysis to help get you started (Adams, 1979).

Let us assume that you and your staff are frustrated at the inefficient ways patients are transported from place to place in your hospital. You decide to discover a new concept of patient transportation. To construct the matrix you need at least three parameters. Let us assume you choose (1) the power source to be used, (2) the devices into which the patient will be put, and (3) the medium in or on which the device will move. Figure 3–1 is the matrix we constructed. Feel free to add additional columns.

Now pick one item at random from each of the three axes and combine them. If, for instance, you got a bed with wheels that ran on people power, you have the conventional gurney—not too helpful. But what if you got a bed on a track that was run by a computer? That *is* a new idea. Now try it several times. List the combinations. Then choose the two most likely new ideas. Choose a name that describes

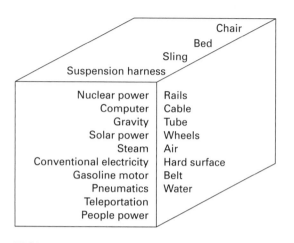

FIGURE 3–1 Three-way matrix.

the new phenomenon. Let your imagination work here. If you got a combination of sling, pneumatic power, and tube, for instance, what could you call it? How about Pneuma-port? or Pneuma-sling? Sling-a-Pat? There are many possibilities.

The next two steps are to verify the concept empirically. In this exercise, verification would need to explore whether or not the technology and the administrative and economic support were available to construct a prototype model. Once the model was constructed, pilot testing would demonstrate its feasibility, efficiency, and effectiveness. The last step is to determine if the prototype fits into existing systems of hospital care or if it requires a whole new system.

This brief exercise may seem very artificial, and it is; but it is one example of concept synthesis and should demonstrate the basic steps for you. Remember, practice makes perfect!

REFERENCES

Adams JL. *Conceptual Blockbusting: A Guide to Better Ideas.* 2nd ed. New York, NY: WW Norton; 1979.

Algase DL, Beck C, Kolanowski A, Berent SK, Richards K, Beattie E. Need-driven dementia-compromised behavior: an alternative view of disruptive behavior. *Am J Alzheimer's Dis.* 1996;11(6):10-19.

Anderson JA, Oinhausen KS. Adolescent self-esteem: a foundational disposition. *Nurs Sci Q.* 1999;12(1):62-67.

Beitz JM. Concept mapping: navigating the learning process. *Nurse Educ.* 1998;23(5):35-41.

Benoliel JQ. Grounded theory and nursing knowledge. *Qual Health Res.* 1996;6:406-428.

Breen J. Transitions in the concept of chronic pain. *Adv Nurs Sci.* 2002;24(4):48-59.

Bunting SM, Russell CK, Gregory DM. Computer monitor. Use of electronic mail (email) for concept synthesis: an international collaborative project. *Qual Health Res.* 1998;8(1):128-135.

Burke SO, Kaufmann, E, Castello EA, Dillon MC. Hazardous secrets and reluctantly taking charge: parenting a child with repeated hospitalizations. *Image.* 1991;23(1):39-45.

Cataldo JK. Hardiness and depression in the institutionalized elderly. *Appl Nurs Res.* 1993;6(2):89-91.

Clunn P. Nurses' assessment of a person's potential for violence: use of grounded theory in developing a nursing diagnosis. In: Kim MJ, McFarland GR, McLane AM, eds. *Classification of Nursing Diagnoses: Proceedings of the Fifth National Conference.* St. Louis, Mo: Mosby; 1984:376-393.

Colling KB. A taxonomy of passive behaviors in people with Alzheimer's disease. *J Nurs Schol.* 2000;32(3):239-244.

Denham SA. Family routines: a structural perspective for viewing family health. *Adv Nurs Sci.* 2002;24(4):60-74.

Dray W. "Explaining what" in history. In: Gardiner P, ed. *Theories of History.* New York, NY: Free Press; 1959.

Eaves YD. A synthesis technique for grounded theory data analysis. *J Adv Nurs.* 2001;35(5):644-653.

Glaser BG. *Basics of Grounded Theory Analysis.* Mill Valley, Calif: Sociology Press; 1992.

Glaser BG. *Theoretical Sensitivity.* Mill Valley, Calif: Sociology Press; 1978.

Glaser BG, Strauss AL. *The Discovery of Grounded Theory: Strategies for Qualitative Research.* Chicago, Ill: Aldine; 1967.

Goldberg B. Connection: an exploration of spirituality in nursing care. *J Adv Nurs.* 1998;27(4):836-842.

Gordon M. *Nursing Diagnosis: Process and Application.* New York, NY: McGraw-Hill; 1982.

Harris CC. Cultural values and the decision to circumcise. *Image.* 1986;18(3):98-104.

Hunt EB. *Concept Learning.* New York, NY: Wiley; 1962.

Kirk J, Miller ML. *Reliability and Validity in Qualitative Research.* Beverly Hills, Calif: Sage Publications; 1986.

Kobasa SC. Personality and resistance to illness. *Am J Commun Psychol.* 1979a;7:413-423.

Kobasa SC. Stressful life events, personality, and health: an inquiry into hardiness. *J Pers Soc Psychol.* 1979b;37:1-11.

Kobasa SC, Hiker RRJ, Maddi SR. Who stays healthy under stress? *J Occup Med.* 1979;21:595-598.

Kolanowski AM. Disturbing behaviors in demented elders: a concept synthesis. *Arch Psychiatr Nurs.* 1995;9(4):188-194.

Lambert CE, Lambert VA. Hardiness: its development and relevance to nursing. *Image.* 1987;19(2):92-95.

Lenz ER, Suppe F, Gift AG, Pugh LC, Milligan RA. Collaborative development of middle-range nursing theories: toward a theory of unpleasant symptoms. *Adv Nurs Sci.* 1995;17(3):1-13.

Moch SD. Health-within-illness: concept development through research and practice. *J Adv Nurs.* 1998;28(2):305-310.

Mullen PD. The potential for grounded theory for health education. In: Glaser BG, ed. *More Grounded Theory Methodology: A Reader.* Mill Valley, Calif: Sociology Press; 1994:127-145.

Nichols PK, Webster A. Hardiness and social support in human immunodeficiency virus. *Appl Nurs Res.* 1993;6(3):132-136.

Oldaker S. Nursing diagnoses among adolescents. In: Hurley ME, ed. *Classification of Nursing Diagnoses: Proceedings of the Sixth National Conference.* St. Louis, Mo: Mosby; 1986:311-318.

Pines M. Psychological hardiness: the role of challenge in health. *Psychol Today.* 1980;14(7):34-42, 98.

Polk LV. Toward a middle-range theory of resilience. *Adv Nurs Sci.* 1997;19(3):1-13.

Ryan-Wenger NM. A taxonomy of children's coping strategies. *Am J Orthopsychiatry.* 1992;62(2):256-263.

Schatzman L, Strauss AL. *Field Research.* Englewood Cliffs, NJ: Prentice Hall; 1973.

Spitzer DR. *Concept Formation and Learning in Early Childhood.* Columbus, OH: Merrill; 1977.

Stern PN. The grounded theory method: its uses and processes. In: Glaser BG, ed. *More Grounded Theory Methodology: A Reader.* Mill Valley, Calif: Sociology Press; 1994:116-126.

Stevenson HW. Concept learning. In: Stevenson HW, ed. *Children's Learning.* New York, NY: Appleton-Century-Crofts; 1972:308-322.

Strauss A, Corbin JM. *Basics of Qualitative Research: Techniques and Procedures for Developing Grounded Theory.* Thousand Oaks, Calif: Sage Publications; 1998.

Wagnild G, Young M. Another look at hardiness. *Image.* 1991;23(4):257-259.

Wendler MC. Using metaphor to explore concept synthesis. *Int J Hum Caring.* 1999;3(1):31-36.

Wilson J. *Thinking with Concepts.* New York, NY: Cambridge University Press; 1963.

ADDITIONAL READINGS

Davitz JR, Davitz LL. *A Guide: Evaluating Research Proposals in the Behavior Sciences.* 2nd ed. New York, NY: Teachers College Press; 1977.

Eakes GC, Burke ML, Hainsworth MA. Middle-range theory of chronic sorrow. *Image.* 1998;30(2):179-184.

Hurley ME, ed. *Classification of Nursing Diagnoses: Proceedings of the Sixth National Conference.* St. Louis, Mo: Mosby; 1986.

Kerlinger FN. *Foundations of Behavioral Research.* 3rd ed. New York, NY: Holt, Rinehart & Winston; 1986.

Klausmeier H. The nature of uses of concepts. In: *Learning and Human Abilities: Educational Psychology.* 4th ed. New York, NY: Harper & Row; 1975:268-298.

Kleinmuntz B, ed. *Concepts and the Structure of Memory.* New York, NY: Wiley; 1967.

Long KA, Weinert C. Rural nursing: developing the theory base. *Scholar Inquiry Nurs Pract.* 1989;3(2):113-127.

Rogge MM. *Development of a Taxonomy of Nursing Interventions: An Analysis of Nursing Care in the American Civil War* [unpublished doctoral dissertation]. Austin: University of Texas; April 1985.

Rosenbaum JN. Self-caring: concept development in nursing. *Recent Adv Nurs.* 1989;24:18-31.

Sandelowski M, Docherty S, Emden C. Qualitative metasynthesis: issues and techniques. *Res Nurs Health.* 1997;20:365-371.

Williams A. A literature review on the concept of intimacy in nursing. *J Adv Nurs.* 2001;33(5):660-667.

4

Concept Derivation

Preliminary Note: *Concept derivation has been one of the less frequently used strate-*
gies in nursing theory development, if one judges by formal citations in articles.
Nonetheless, its informal use is no doubt more widespread. Reasoning by analogy or
metaphor is a powerful experience during creative work. It is commonplace when try-
ing to express novel ideas to look to other areas of inquiry for insight and inspiration.
In presenting this chapter on concept derivation, we attempt to give the reader some ex-
plicit guidance in how to derive concepts that may enrich their theorizing within prac-
tice, teaching, or research.

DEFINITION AND DESCRIPTION

The basis of concept derivation lies in an analogy between phenomena in two
fields or areas of inquiry. The process of concept derivation builds on the earlier
work of Maccia (1963) and Maccia and Maccia (1963). By looking to a defined
source or parent field for an analog to aid in developing a new field of interest, concepts in the new field may be derived. Further, by redefining concepts from the
parent field to fit the new field, a new set of concepts is created. Thus, the newly
defined concepts no longer rely on the parent field for meaning. The parent field
may reside either within the broader discipline of nursing or in other disciplines.

The strategy of concept derivation is applicable where a meaningful analogy
can be made between one field that is conceptually defined and another that is not.
Expressed more precisely, concept derivation consists of moving a concept (C_1)
from one field of inquiry (F_1) to another field (F_2). In the process of transposing a
concept, it is necessary that the concept (C_1) be redefined as a new concept (C_2)
that fits the new field of inquiry (F_2). This process is diagrammed in Figure 4–1.
Thus C_1 leads to C_2, but F_1 and F_2 are *not* the same. Redefinition of C_1 results in a
concept (C_2) that is based on but different from C_1.

At first glance concept derivation might appear to be a mechanical process.
Nonetheless, creativity and imagination are required. First of all, a theorist must
select a parent field (F_1) with concepts that bear an analogy to the new field or area
of inquiry. To grasp the analogous nature of two fields may require first taking the

52

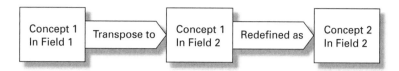

FIGURE 4–1   Process of concept derivation.

time for immersion in the potential parent field of inquiry. In some cases, concepts from the natural sciences have been extended into the social and behavioral sciences. For example, concepts such as "system" from biology and "energy" from physics are common in both the social and behavioral sciences as well as nursing. There is no rule, however, about where one may find a rich conceptual perspective for concept derivation. Insight of the theorist is needed.

Creativity and imagination are needed for a second reason: meaningful redefinition of the concepts when they are transposed into the new field of inquiry. Redefining is more than merely assigning a slightly modified definition to a word. The type of redefinition that occurs in productive concept derivation requires that the derived concepts be linked to the new field (F_2) by definitions that result in truly innovative ways of looking at phenomena in F_2. One of the most productive uses of concept derivation results when a new taxonomy or typology of phenomena in F_2 is derived. A new taxonomy or typology provides not only a new vocabulary for classifying phenomena in F_2 but, more importantly, new ways of looking at F_2. An important typology introduced into nursing was derived by Roy (Roy & Roberts, 1981, p. 55). Using Helson's concepts of focal, contextual, and residual stimuli from psychophysics, Roy redefined these concepts within nursing to form a typology of factors related to adaptation levels of persons (pp. 53–55). This derivation process is presented in Figure 4–2.

Concept derivation is more than simply applying a concept in unchanged form to a phenomenon where it has not been previously used. The meaning of the concept must be developed and changed to fit a new phenomenon. For example, assume that the concept "role change" has not been previously applied to the transition from in-hospital patient to out-patient status. Assume further that role change may be applied to the transition in patient status without any change in the meaning of the concept of role change. Although the application of that concept to transition in patient status may be scientifically interesting, it is not a true case of concept derivation because role change was simply linked to a new phenomenon to which it already had relevance and meaning. Role change thus was not used as a metaphor or analogy, but rather its meaning was left intact.

PURPOSE AND USES

The purpose of concept derivation is to generate new ways of thinking about and looking at some phenomenon. It provides a new vocabulary for an area of inquiry by

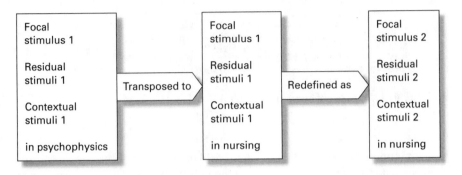

FIGURE 4–2   Concept derivation from Helson's to Roy's concepts.

relying on an analogous or metaphorical relationship between two phenomena: one defined and known, one undefined and under exploration. By relying on a parent field (F_1) for ways of talking about and understanding another (F_2), the concept development process can be accelerated compared to slower methods such as concept synthesis, which relies on analysis of observations and data in concept development.

There are two situations in which concept derivation may be particularly useful: (1) in potential fields or areas in where no concept development has yet taken place; and (2) in fields in which currently existing concepts have contributed little to advancing inquiry about the phenomenon of interest, either in practical or theoretical terms. In other words, the field is "stuck."

It is not uncommon for nurses to encounter new situations in which little existing conceptual work has been done, for example, dealing with patients in their 10th decade who have no living relatives except grandchildren and great-grandchildren. Existing concepts about parent–child relationships may simply not apply to understanding these skipped-generational family relationships. In such situations concept derivation may be useful. In another instance, Brauer (2001) reported using concept derivation in concept development related to functioning among persons with rheumatoid arthritis.

Alternatively, concepts in existence may simply become outmoded, hence more innovative ways of classifying the phenomena in a field may be needed. For example, the traditional concepts that divided areas of nursing practice into medical, surgical, obstetrical, pediatric, and psychiatric nursing are less relevant today than in the past. These divisions are less useful now as more and more is known about how developmental, environmental, and psychological factors interact with the human body to produce disease and health in people across the life span. Thus, a new perspective for classifying nursing specialties and their respective knowledge domains is needed. Concept derivation may be helpful in constructing a more relevant classification system. In another example, inquiry about "dyspnea" as a subjective experience was advanced by using dimensions of pain as an analog to dimensions of dyspnea (Lenz , Suppe, Gift, Pugh, & Milligan, 1995).

PROCEDURES FOR CONCEPT DERIVATION

Four basic steps or phases comprise the concept derivation strategy. Whereas some of these steps in actual practice may occur simultaneously, we present them in logical sequence to facilitate clarity. Further, users of this strategy may find as they proceed that they need to return to preceding steps to clarify or validate their work at an earlier step. This is especially likely to happen as users move from an orientation phase, that is, getting familiar with their topic of interest, to the intense working phase. We underscore these points so that readers are not misled. Concept derivation is an efficient strategy for concept development, but to carry it out adequately is not necessarily a quick, mechanical process.

1.   First, the concept developer needs to become thoroughly familiar with existing literature related to the topic of interest. This involves not only reading the literature but also critiquing the level and usefulness of existing concept development found there. If the existing literature on your topic of interest is lacking in relevant concepts, or if concepts exist but they have ceased to stimulate growth of understanding about the topic, then concept derivation may be suitable as a theory development strategy.

2.   Examine other fields for new ways of looking at the topic of interest. Read widely in both related and dissimilar fields. Because you cannot know in advance exactly where the most fruitful analogies will be found, it is advisable to begin by casting a broad net at first. From a practical standpoint, it is important not to rush this step; frequently the analogies surface or become apparent at unexpected times and places. Because this step relies to some extent on creative insight, it can be facilitated by maintaining a relaxed, patient attitude and not trying to force an immediate solution.

3.   Choose a parent concept or set of concepts from another field to use in the derivation process. The parent–field concepts should offer a new and insightful way of viewing the topic of interest. For example, suppose you were puzzled by some unexpected findings about inconsistencies within hospital workers under stress. You might turn to the field of submarine design for an analogy to understand the "compartmentalizing" that seemed to be occurring. The choice of a parent field may come in a "flash" or may be the result of a careful fitting process between the new and the parent field (Lenz et al., 1995).

4.   Last, redefine the concept or set of concepts from the parent field in terms of the topic of interest. In the example mentioned in step 3, the hospital workers' inconsistencies were conceptualized as the "submarine syndrome," which was defined as closing off areas in which an employee was experiencing stress so that these did not interfere with other areas of functioning—analogous to efforts to prevent sinking the submarine. Furthermore, if a *set* of concepts are being redefined in terms of the topic of interest, these can provide a preliminary taxonomy for describing the basic types that comprise the topic of interest. Once a preliminary set of definitions has been made, check these out with colleagues familiar with the topic of interest. Any constructive criticism received, even though momentarily painful, can be very helpful in further refining the initial work. Be sure to give yourself a pat on the back at this point!

A classic illustration of the process of concept derivation is contained in Sameroff's work on levels of parental thinking about the parent–child relationship (Sameroff, 1980, pp. 348–352). Sameroff, an expert in child development, began with a working familiarity of literature on human development and family relationships. Sameroff was searching for a new way of understanding parental thought processes that might explain differences in parental childrearing behaviors. He reviewed existing concepts relevant to understanding parental thinking: parental attitudes and expectations and social norms. These concepts in themselves provided only limited ways of understanding parental thinking. In sum, a new perspective was needed. Sameroff was interested in "the level of abstraction utilized by parents to understand development" (p. 349). He turned to the groundbreaking work of the French psychologist Piaget (1963), in which stages of cognitive development in children were elaborated. Sameroff identified an analogy between cognitive development in children and parental thinking:

> *Research on the cognitive development of the child has shown that the infant must go through a number of stages before achieving the logical thought processes that characterize adulthood. Similarly, parents may use different levels in thinking about their relationship with the child. (p. 349)*

Based on Piaget's four stages of cognitive development (sensorimotor, preoperational, concrete operational, and formal operational), Sameroff proposed by analogy four levels of parental thinking. Briefly, in Piaget's classic work on the sensorimotor stage the advent of language marks a stage in which cognition is tied to actions, with learning rooted in the senses and manipulation. With passage into the next stage, the preoperational, the child uses images and symbols in addition to actions in cognitive processes, but objects are understood in terms of single methods of classification, for example, size. Advancing to the concrete operational stage allows the child to think in terms of logical operations or rules, such as equivalence and serialization—for example, grouping objects in a series by size. In Piaget's final stage of formal operations the child's logical operations move beyond concrete realities to abstract possibilities that may be proposed and evaluated (Biehler, 1971; Mussen, Conger, & Kagan, 1980; Piaget, 1963).

In his work, Sameroff proposed four analogous levels of parental thinking: symbiotic, categorical, compensatory, and perspectivistic (see Figure 4–3). Parents who respond to the child from the symbiotic level act on a here-and-now basis. Parents do not separate the child's or infant's responses from their own actions. At the categorical level parents see themselves as separate from the child. The child's behavior stems from traits or characteristics of the child; for example, the child is stubborn. Parents who view the child from a compensatory level see the child's behavior as age related—for instance, the child is stubborn because he or she is a toddler. At the perspectivistic level, parents see the child's behavior "as stemming from individual experiences in specific environments. If those experiences had been different, the child's characteristics would be different" (Sameroff, 1980,

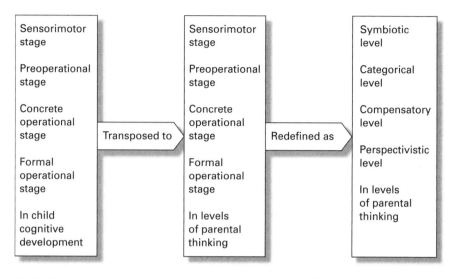

FIGURE 4–3   Concept derivation from Piaget's to Sameroff's concepts.

p. 352). Interestingly, Sameroff found that the majority of parents he studied functioned at the categorical level.

Looking back at Sameroff's process, his expertise in the child development field allowed him to complete the first two steps of concept derivation with ease. He knew the literature and was able to critique the utility of existing concepts in the field. This expertise also made readily available to him alternative perspectives needed in deriving concepts about parental thinking levels and also led to selecting Piaget's work as most promising. He then proceeded to flesh out the parental levels of thinking that were analogous to Piaget's stages. In the final step of concept derivation, Sameroff transposed Piaget's concepts and redefined them in ways relevant to parental thinking. He also created new labels for his four stages so that the terms in his new framework better fit the parenting phenomenon.

An example of concept derivation in nursing may be found in the work of Braun, Wykle, and Cowling (1988), who derived the concept of "failure to thrive in older persons." Noting the phenomenon of weight loss among some institutionalized elderly, they proposed that "failure to thrive among elderly persons may, perhaps, mirror the [already established] pediatric phenomenon" of failure to thrive (p. 809). To further develop the concept of failure to thrive with the elderly, a careful review of literature was done to identify similarities and differences between pediatric and geriatric symptoms and origins. They concluded that pediatric failure to thrive is "a global concept with multiple possible . . . etiologies" and includes weight loss and developmental and depressive symptoms (p. 811). In elderly people, the concept may be "viewed as a broad symptom complex originating, perhaps, from varied physiological, psychological, or combined sources" manifested in weight loss, physical and cognitive decline, and depressive symptoms such as hopelessness (p. 812).

Braun and colleagues' (1988) derivation builds on the similarity between some of the manifestations of weight loss noted across these two developmental stages. Although not identical phenomena, the parent field (pediatric literature) was used to structure the development of the concept of failure to thrive among the elderly. However, the concepts are different in that pediatric failure to thrive is associated with growth and developmental retardation, whereas in elderly people the concept represents a process of decline in weight and functioning.

Several things should be kept in mind in applying concept derivation to nursing. First, because the concerns of nurses may overlap with those of other health professions, the first step of concept derivation need not be limited to nursing literature. Medical, educational, developmental, and social work literature, to mention only a few, may be relevant to developing a sense of extant concepts about the topic of interest. Should concepts from these related fields seem adequate, there is no need to proceed any further. In turn, if an extensive search of literature shows that related fields have not attended to the topic of interest, or if the conceptual work elsewhere seems limited, then concept derivation in nursing may benefit these other fields as well.

Second, as noted earlier, there is no rule about where to look for rich analogies or metaphors for nursing phenomena. In addition to fields of inquiry in nursing, the natural sciences (physics, zoology, chemistry) and behavioral sciences as well as applied areas such as law, engineering, and education may be considered. Discussions with nursing colleagues as well as experts in other fields may be useful in identifying potentially useful parent fields from which to derive concepts.

Third, theorists should not be impatient in selecting a promising set of concepts from which to derive concepts for nursing phenomena. Frequently, assimilation or incubation time is needed to see the fit between two fields of study. This type of insight typically comes in "a flash" that may be preceded by a period of frustrating lack of progress.

Fourth, the final step of concept derivation, redefining the concepts in terms of the phenomena in the field of interest, may be laborious. Definitions may need to be redone several times before a final satisfactory outcome is achieved. Setting aside the work for brief periods may be helpful in producing the new and creative perspective desired. Critically judging the merits of one's work prematurely may also stifle creativity. The theorist should remain patient but persistent.

ADVANTAGES AND LIMITATIONS

Concept derivation as a strategy has the advantage of letting the theorist avoid beginning from scratch. The use of concepts from another field speeds along the creative process. Indeed, Maccia (1963) has suggested that the perspective that concept derivation employs may underlie sources of theory development in general.

Two limitations to concept derivation as a theory development strategy should be borne in mind. First, although the derived concepts may provide useful labels, concepts alone are limited in their scientific usefulness. In themselves, concepts do not provide explanations, predictions, or control of phenomena. Only relational statements and theories have this potential (see Chapter 2). Development of concepts, however, can be the first stage in development of statements and theories. Concepts may label the dimensions of a phenomenon, but more is needed to achieve the larger goals of science and practice.

Second, despite the fact that a concept (C_1) from the parent field (F_1) has been useful in that field, a concept derived from it (C_2) may not automatically be equally so. Unfortunately, being well born does not guarantee success. Thus, the scientific utility of a derived concept is unknown until it is tested in practice and research (see Chapter 12). Uncertainty about the scientific usefulness of new ideas is not limited to concept derivation as a strategy. There is risk endemic in proposing any new idea. Until ideas are tested, their value remains unknown.

UTILIZING THE RESULTS OF CONCEPT DERIVATION

Concepts developed through the derivation strategy may be used in at least two ways in research and theory development: (1) derived concepts can provide working concepts for use in clinical work such as nursing diagnosis development; and (2) derived concepts can provide preliminary classification schemes of nursing phenomena for use in further research, theory development, and clinical practice. In these uses it is important to determine if the concepts derived have empirical validity in the new field.

To test the validity of derived diagnostic concepts, readers are referred to the classic methodology literature in the field of nursing diagnosis (e.g., Gordon & Sweeney, 1979). In research and theory development, derived concepts should be reassessed for their utility in describing phenomena in ways that further the aims of a field of study and that pull together the findings of relevant research. Where derived concepts delineate new phenomena in need of systematic measurement, they may be used as the base for tool development (see Waltz, Strickland, & Lenz [1991] on operationalizing nursing concepts).

Moreover, concept derivation can be used as an instructional heuristic in the teaching–learning process. When introducing unfamiliar concepts to students, analogs can facilitate concept introduction. Such application of concept derivation requires that useful analogs be available and already understood by students.

SUMMARY

The strategy of concept derivation employs an analogy or metaphor to transpose concepts from one field of inquiry to another. There are no exact rules for selecting a field from which to derive concepts. Concept derivation is suited to topics of interest in which there is no extant concept development or in which existing concepts have become stagnant. The steps in concept derivation include becoming familiar with and critiquing existing literature on a topic, searching other fields for conceptual perspectives, choosing a promising set of concepts from which to derive new concepts, and then generating new concepts by analogy from the parent field. The strategy of concept derivation may speed up the concept development process. The strategy is limited by the level of theory achieved and the uncertainty about the ultimate usefulness of the derived concepts.

PRACTICE EXERCISE

You may try out the steps of the concept derivation process using the practice exercise that follows. Because it is not feasible to do each step completely, we will assume that preparatory steps have been completed already to facilitate the exercise.

First, let's start by assuming that you are interested in a new way of understanding nurse–patient communication in primary care settings. Let's also assume that after an extensive review of literature on nurse–patient communication your suspicion is confirmed that the literature lacks innovative concepts relevant to nurse–patient communication in primary care settings. After searching the behavioral sciences and finding little that seems promising, you happen to talk with a geographer at a social function. He is discussing the concepts that underlie the design and uses of maps. During the course of the conversation, you see a striking analogy between the map concepts and idea of nurse–patient communication in primary care. You see the patient as a "traveler" and the nurse as a source of "travel information" in getting to a "destination."

In this exercise, take out a map of your state. List the kinds of information the map provides a traveler. List how you use a map as you travel between two cities in your state. List the different reasons you might be traveling and how this might affect what you refer to on the map. Review these lists thoroughly. Now select the key ideas from these lists that seem to you to describe the ways a traveler uses a map to get to a destination. Now think of the patient and nurse in a primary care setting. Transfer your key ideas (i.e., concepts) about the ways a traveler uses a map to the primary care setting. Use these key ideas to think about nurse–patient communication. When you get a feel for these key ideas in the primary care setting, jot down short definitions that describe the concepts in terms of nurse–patient communication. Do not worry yet about whether your definitions and concepts make sense. Set aside your work for a while. Look at your key concepts and definitions again. Clarify any fuzzy wording or ideas. Now try out your ideas on some colleagues who will give constructive criticism. From their reactions, further refine your concepts and definitions.

Bear in mind, there is no one "right" set of concepts or definitions that you should have derived. If you had had a colleague simultaneously do this same exercise, that person's concepts and definitions would probably be somewhat different from yours. For comparison purposes, two examples of concepts that we derived by this exercise are presented in Table 4–1. In Example 2, the defining characteristics of the derived concepts are also provided. You may find that the concepts and definitions that you derived are more interesting than the ones we presented!

TABLE 4–1   TWO EXAMPLES OF DERIVED CONCEPTS

Parent Field: Informational Functions of Maps for Travelers	New Field of Interest: Informational Functions of Primary Care Nurses
Example 1. Parent Concepts	Example 1. Derived Concepts
1. Direction	1. Orientation
2. Points of interest	2. Facilities available
3. Alternate routes	3. Alternates for diagnosis and treatment
4. Mileage estimates	4. Duration of care
5. Geographic reference points	5. Reference points for progress
6. Destination	6. Goal of care
Example 2. Parent Concepts and Defining Qualities	Example 2. Derived Concepts and Defining Qualities
1. Business travel—for a specific purpose	1. Focused care—care of a specific problem
1.1 Efficient travel pace	1.1 Rapid attention to presenting problem
1.2 Direct route on main thoroughfares	1.2 Focus of attention on presenting problem
1.3 Specific information on access points on route	1.3 Specific information about time and place of treatments
1.4 Reliable accommodations	1.4 Reliable personnel and facilities
1.5 Time frame limited to specific business objective	1.5 Time frame for care determined by presenting problem
2. Pleasure travel—travel for recreation and growth	2. Revitalization care—care for health promotion
2.1 Leisurely pace of travel	2.1 Careful consideration to patient concerns and questions
2.2 Scenic routes	2.2 Attention to overall health status
2.3 Alternate access points for possible side trips	2.3 Information about health promotion alternatives
2.4 Pleasurable accommodations	2.4 Competent and humanistic care
2.5 Time frame negotiable based on wishes	2.5 Time frame negotiated based on health promotion needs and wants

REFERENCES

Biehler RF. *Psychology Applied to Teaching.* Boston, Mass: Houghton Mifflin; 1971.

Brauer DJ. Common patterns of person-environment interaction in persons with rheumatoid arthritis. *West J Nurs Res.* 2001;23:414-430.

Braun JV, Wykle MH, Cowling WR. Failure to thrive in older persons. *Gerontologist.* 1988; 28:809-812.

Gordon M, Sweeney MA. Methodological problems and issues in identifying and standardizing nursing diagnoses. *Adv Nurs Sci.* 1979;2(1):1-15.

Lenz ER, Suppe F, Gift AG, Pugh LC, Milligan RA. Collaborative development of middle-range nursing theories: toward a theory of unpleasant symptoms. *Adv Nurs Sci.* 1995; 17(3):1-13.

Maccia ES. Ways of inquiring. In: Maccia ES, Maccia GS, Jewett RS, eds. *Construction of Educational Theory Models.* Washington, DC: Office of Education, US Dept of Health, Education, and Welfare, Cooperative Research Project No. 1632; 1963;1-13.

Maccia ES, Maccia GS. The way of educational theorizing through models. In: Maccia ES, Maccia GS, Jewett RE, eds. *Construction of Educational Theory Models.* Washington, DC: Office of Education, US Dept of Health, Education, and Welfare, Cooperative Research Project No. 1632; 1963;30-45.

Mussen PH, Conger JJ, Kagan J. *Essentials of Child Development and Personality.* Philadelphia, Penn: Harper & Row; 1980.

Piaget J. *Psychology of Intelligence.* Paterson, NJ: Littlefield, Adams & Co; 1963.

Roy C, Roberts SL. *Theory Construction in Nursing: An Adaptation Model.* Englewood Cliffs, NJ: Prentice Hall; 1981.

Sameroff AJ. Issues in early reproductive and caretaking risk: review and current status. In: Sawin DB, Hawkins RCB, Walker LO, Penticuff JH, eds. *Exceptional Infant.* Vol. 4. *Psychosocial Risks in Infant–Environment Transactions.* New York, NY: Brunner/Mazel; 1980; 343-359.

Waltz CF, Strickland OL, Lenz ER. *Measurement in Nursing Research.* 2nd ed. Philadelphia, Penn: Davis; 1991.

5

Concept Analysis

Preliminary Note: There has been a lot of concept analysis work since the last edition of this book. What a great thing to see! It is encouraging to note that nurse scholars and clinicians are beginning to take nursing vocabularies seriously and to make the effort to clearly define the concepts of interest to them. The only way we will be able to demonstrate the evidence base for our practice is to be able to first describe the phenomena in a measurable or at least communicable way. Concept analysis allows the theorist, researcher, or clinician to come to grips with the various possibilities within the concept of interest—to "get inside" the concept and see how it works. It is a challenging activity but provides an enormous insight into the phenomenon of interest.

DEFINITION AND DESCRIPTION

Examining the structure and function of a concept is the purpose of concept analysis (see Chapter 2). Concepts contain within themselves the attributes or characteristics that make them unique from other concepts. Thus, we speak of concepts as containing defining characteristics or attributes that permit us to decide which phenomena match the concept and which do not. Concepts are mental constructions; they are our attempts to order our environmental stimuli. Concepts, therefore, represent categories of information that contain defining attributes. Concept analysis is a formal, linguistic exercise to determine those defining attributes. The analysis itself must be rigorous and precise, but the end product is always tentative. The reasons for this tentativeness stem from the fact that two people will often come up with somewhat different attributes for the same concept in their analyses, and from the fact that scientific and general knowledge changes so quickly that what is "true" today is "not true" tomorrow.

Contributing to the tentativeness of concepts is that they also change over time—often slowly, but occasionally very quickly. Therefore, anyone undertaking concept analysis should be aware of the dynamic quality of ideas and the words that express those ideas. Concepts are not carved in stone. Analysts change over time as well. Therefore, their understanding of the concept may also change over time. This is one reason why concept analyses should never be viewed as a "finished product." The best one can hope for from a concept analysis is to capture the critical elements of it at the current moment in time. However, this is not to imply that trying to determine the defining attributes of a concept of interest is futile—far from it.

Concept analysis encourages communication. If we are precise about carefully defining the attributes of the concepts we use in theory development and in research, we will make it far easier to promote understanding among our colleagues about the phenomena being discussed.

PURPOSE AND USES

Concept analysis is a process of examining the basic elements of a concept. If we know "what counts" when we describe a concept, it helps us to distinguish that concept from ones that are similar to but not the same as that concept. It allows us to distinguish the likeness and unlikeness between concepts. By breaking a concept into its simpler elements, it is easier to determine its internal structure. Because we have already said in Chapter 2 that a concept is expressed by a word or a term in language (Reynolds, 1971), an analysis of a concept must, perforce, be an analysis of the descriptive word and its use. Concept analysis is ultimately only a careful examination and description of a word or term and its uses in the language coupled with an explanation of how it is "like" and "not like" other related words or terms. We are concerned with both actual and possible uses of words that convey concept meanings.

Concept analysis can be useful in refining ambiguous concepts in a theory. It also helps clarify those overused or vague concepts that are prevalent in nursing practice so that everyone who subsequently uses the term will be speaking of the same thing. Concept analysis results in a precise operational definition that by its very nature increases the validity of the construct; that is, it will accurately reflect its theoretical base. The results of concept analysis yield to the theorist or investigator a basic understanding of the underlying attributes of the concepts. This helps to clearly define the problem and to allow the investigator or theorist to construct hypotheses that accurately reflect the relationships between the concepts. The results of concept analysis are also very useful in constructing research instruments or interview guides prior to doing research.

In a classic textbook, Nunnally (1978) has spoken to the need for careful conceptual development for research instruments. The results of concept analysis—the operational definition, list of defining attributes, and antecedents—can provide the scientist with an excellent beginning for a new tool or an excellent way to evaluate an old one. To begin a new tool, items could be constructed to reflect each of the defining attributes. Questions could be constructed to determine whether proposed antecedents occurred. With careful psychometric testing, the new tool could be useful for continuing research by interested scientists. The results of concept analysis are also useful in evaluating existing instruments. The instruments to be used in a research project could be examined in light of the results of the concept analysis to determine if the instruments accurately reflect the defining attributes of the relevant concepts.

Developing standardized language to describe nursing practice is another primary use of concept analysis. In many cases, the terms to describe nursing diagnoses, interventions, and outcomes have been developed consensually or in practice settings without thoroughly considering the theoretical issues relating to assigning names to clients' problems or to the interventions we provide nor to the outcomes we can reasonably expect (Carlson-Catalano et al., 1998; Gamel, Grypdonck, Hengeveld, & Davis, 2001; Whitley, 1995). Conducting a thorough concept analysis for any potential diagnosis, intervention, or outcome would greatly facilitate taxonomic work and would thoroughly ground nursing language in the pertinent theoretical and research literature. Each nursing diagnosis, intervention, and outcome should be treated as a separate concept and be analyzed independently. For instance, most nursing diagnoses are written with three components—the health problem, the etiology, and the defining signs and symptoms (Gordon, 1982). These three components closely parallel the results of concept analysis—antecedents (etiology), defining characteristics (defining signs and symptoms), and operational definition (health problem). It seems reasonable to suggest using the two processes iteratively to improve our taxonomies and contribute to theory development simultaneously.

The method we describe below is only one of several methods available for concept analysis. We feel it is the easiest to understand and master, especially for beginners.

PROCEDURES FOR CONCEPT ANALYSIS

We have modified and simplified Wilson's (1963) classic concept analysis procedure so there are only 8 instead of 11 steps. We believe that the 8 steps are sufficient to capture the essence of the process. The steps are as follows:

1. Select a concept.
2. Determine the aims or purposes of analysis.
3. Identify all uses of the concept that you can discover.
4. Determine the defining attributes.
5. Identify a model case.
6. Identify borderline, related, contrary, invented, and illegitimate cases.
7. Identify antecedents and consequences.
8. Define empirical referents.

Although we will discuss the steps in concept analysis as if they were sequential, in fact they are iterative. The mental activities of a concept analysis often require that some revision be made in an earlier step because of information or ideas arising from a later one. This is to be expected. The iterative nature of the process results in a much cleaner, more precise analysis.

Select a Concept

Concept selection should be done with care. It is best to choose a concept in which you are already interested, one that is associated with your work, or one that has always "bothered" you. This first step is often the hardest because you may have several concepts that interest you. How do you choose just one? Generally, concept selection should reflect the topic or area of greatest interest to you. Our advice is to choose the one that is most critical to your needs. Is there one concept on which everything else depends? Is there a concept that is critical to doing the next step in your research? If so, this is the concept you should choose first. Wilson (1963) describes this process as isolating the concept—that is, examining the significance of the concept in its various contexts, boundaries, and relevance to your own work.

Choose a concept that is manageable, especially if this is your first concept analysis. It is important to avoid primitive terms that can be defined only by giving examples. It is equally important to avoid "umbrella" terms that are so broad they may encompass several meanings and confuse the analysis.

Unexplored concepts can be either fruitful avenues of exploration or linguistic traps. Unexplored concepts can be found in nursing practice, can be generated from nursing research studies, or can be drawn from a theory that is as yet incomplete or that has concepts that are unclear. Analysis of one of these can be very helpful in expanding your thinking. However, by their nature (unexplored) they may lead you down a path that you do not want to tread or that takes you in the wrong direction. If this is so, you may want to consider abandoning the analysis and choosing a more relevant concept.

The bottom line is that you should choose a concept that is important and useful to your research program or to further theoretical developments in your area of interest. Choosing a trivial concept or one that does not contribute significantly to knowledge development about your phenomenon of concern is an exercise in futility and a waste of your valuable time.

Determine the Aims of Analysis

To determine the aims or purposes of the analysis is the next step. This second step helps focus attention on exactly what use you intend to make of the results of your effort. It essentially answers the question: "Why am I doing this analysis?"

It is very important to decide for yourself, in advance, why you are interested in conducting a concept analysis. Write it down and keep it handy during the analysis. This definition of purpose is useful if, as you begin to determine the defining attributes, you discover several dissimilar uses of the concept. The selection you make regarding which specific use of the concept you will choose should reflect the aims of the analysis.

Distinguishing between the normal, ordinary language usage of the concept and the scientific usage of the same concept might be the aim of your analysis. Others might be to clarify the meaning of an existing concept, to develop an operational definition, or to add to existing theory. There are other possible purposes. Whatever the purpose is for your analysis, keep it clearly in mind as you work.

In our analysis of attachment at the end of this chapter, you will see that because we were interested in the concept of attachment as it applied to mothers and babies, we had to distinguish between animate and inanimate instances of attachment. If our aim had not been related to animate attachment, we might have made different decisions about how to proceed when we realized there would be differences.

Identify Uses of the Concept

Using dictionaries, thesauruses, colleagues, and available literature, identify as many uses of the concept as you can find. At this initial stage do not limit yourself to only one aspect of the concept. You must consider all uses of the term. Do not limit your search to just nursing or medical literature as this may bias your understanding of the true nature of the concept. Ignoring the physical aspects of a concept and focusing only on the psychosocial, for instance, may deprive you of a great deal of valuable information. Remember to include both implicit as well as explicit uses of the concept. Extensive reading in as many different sources as possible is invaluable.

This review of literature helps you support or validate your ultimate choices of the defining attributes. For instance, if you were examining the concept of "coping," you would discover that not only are there psychological uses for the term but there are also copings on buildings, coping saws, a method of trimming a falcon's beak called coping, and a coping that is an ecclesiastical garment similar to a cloak. All of these uses of the term must be included in your final analysis.

Failing to identify, or worse, ignoring some uses of a concept may result in an analysis that severely limits the usefulness of the outcome. A few years ago, one of our students was analyzing the concept "presence" as it relates to the care of hospitalized children. In the initial phase, the student reported many positive uses of the concept but none that were negative. When other students mentioned things such as "evil presence" or "presence of a hostile army on the border," the student was reluctant to consider those aspects of presence. Yet, in the final analysis, one critical attribute of the nurse's "presence" with a hospitalized child turned out to be the potential for threat engendered in the presence of the nurse. Smith's (2001) excellent article is recommended, along with the commentary by Chase (2001) for a thorough and interesting review of the state of the science about the concept of presence.

Once you have identified all the usages of the concept, both ordinary and scientific, you may have to decide whether to continue to consider all aspects of the concept or only those pertinent to the scientific use. We generally feel that when possible you should continue to consider all aspects of the concept usage because that is likely to yield richer meanings. However, at times that will clearly be impractical or unhelpful. In these cases, use the aims of your analysis to guide your decision making.

During your review of the literature and in the process of collecting instances of concept use, you will find other instances that are similar or related to the concept being analyzed but are not quite the "real thing." Keep a list of these instances. They will be helpful to you when you begin to construct borderline or related cases.

Determine the Defining Attributes

Determining the defining attributes is the heart of concept analysis. The effort is to try to show the cluster of attributes that are the most frequently associated with the concept and that allow the analyst the broadest insight into the concept. As you examine as many of the different instances of a concept as you can find, make notes of the characteristics of the concept that appear over and over again. This list of characteristics, called defining characteristics or defining attributes, functions very much like the criteria for making differential diagnoses in medicine. That is, they help you and others name the occurrence of a specific phenomenon as differentiated from another similar or related one.

The defining attributes are not immutable. They may change as your understanding of the concept improves. They may change slightly over time if the concept changes. Or they may change when used in a different context than the one under study.

If, when you have gathered all the instances of a concept, there are a large number of possible meanings, then a decision is clearly necessary regarding which will be the most useful and which will provide you the greatest help in relation to the aims of your analysis. You may decide to choose more than one meaning and continue analyzing using several meanings. For example, in the analysis of the concept of "attachment" at the end of this chapter we found that attachment can occur in both animate and inanimate forms. We chose to examine which attributes were common to both kinds and then to continue our analysis further to include the specific defining attributes for animate attachment because our area of interest was in mother–infant attachment (Avant, 1979). Consideration of the social or nursing care context in which the concept is to be used may be important in your decision as it was to us in the example. The final decision is up to you.

The three characteristics that seemed to be most obvious among all those divergent uses of the term "coping," for instance, were (1) the attribute of covering something—an action, a cape, a window, a beak; (2) the attribute of protection—one's psyche, the garment under the cape, the flowers under the window; and (3) the attribute of adjusting or rebalancing. We decided that the idea of the coping saw was not relevant to the general concept because it does not reflect any of the three attributes that occur in all the other instances we found. We will use this, in fact, as the example of an "illegitimate" case later in the analysis—one in which the term is used incorrectly in relation to its generally accepted meaning.

In Ellis-Stoll and Popkess-Vawter's (1998) study, the defining attributes of empowerment were identified as mutual participation, active listening, and individualized knowledge acquisition. The model case presented regarded James, a postcoronary bypass patient in rehabilitation. In the model case, the defining attributes were clearly observable. This demonstration of the defining characteristics is one of the principal reasons for the model case.

Identify Model Case(s)

A model case is an example of the use of the concept that demonstrates all the defining attributes of the concept. That is, the model case should be a pure case of the concept, a paradigmatic example, or a pure exemplar. Basically, the model case is one that we are absolutely sure is an instance of the concept. Wilson (1963) suggests that the model case is one in which the analyst can say, "Well, if that isn't an example of it, then nothing is." The model case can come first in your analysis, may be developed simultaneously with the attributes, or may emerge after the attributes are tentatively determined.

Model cases may be actual examples from real life, found in the literature, or even constructed by you. The model case may be a nursing example or not. That depends on you. Sometimes using a nursing model case helps you understand the concept, but sometimes it obscures your ability to be objective about the concept meanings. You must find the examples and set them up in such a way as to be useful to your analysis. Some concepts lend themselves more easily than others to this effort.

When a concept is familiar to you, the model case often comes first in your analysis. Because you are familiar with it, you know about instances of it. Thus, you can compare your experience to the defining attributes you have found for the concept. Do they match? If not, why not? What things are different, missing, or additional in either the defining attributes or the model case that makes them inconsistent? The answers to these questions can help you refine the defining attributes. Wilson (1963) calls this back-and-forth examination of cases and defining attributes an internal dialogue. It is a kind of constant comparative reflection that takes place while you are actively working on the analysis. It helps you come to grips with the internal structure of the concept and hence to clarify its meaning and context.

However, the internal dialogue can take you only so far. At some point you will want to think aloud about your analysis. It is often helpful and sometimes necessary to seek out a thoughtful colleague or two who can listen with a fresh ear as you talk through your examples. If there are flaws or errors you haven't seen, it is likely that someone else can spot them for you. At times, the best you will be able to do may be a little fuzzy at the edges, especially if the concept has several synonyms or related concepts that overlap the concept of interest. Don't despair. The effort here is to try to keep the case as paradigmatic as possible.

In our coping example, for instance, the model case was stated as follows:

> *A young woman is walking along a street wearing high heels and a silk dress. On her briefcase is a pouch with an umbrella in it. As she walks, it begins to rain heavily. She takes out her umbrella and raises it. She begins to run, but stumbles. She stops, removes her shoes quickly, and resumes running to the nearest shelter.*

This model case includes all three of the critical attributes, covering, protection, and rebalancing. There are several other examples, or cases, of coping that could have been used instead. We tried to use one that was simple and commonplace for demonstration.

Identify Additional Cases

Examining other cases is another part of the internal dialogue. Teasing out the defining attributes that most closely represent the concept of interest may be difficult because they may overlap with some related concepts. Examining cases that are not exactly the same as the concept of interest but are similar to it or contrary to it in some ways will help you make better judgments about which defining attributes or characteristics have the best "fit." We will discuss several types of cases that have proved useful in the past. The basic purpose for these cases is to help you decide what "counts" as a defining attribute for the concept of interest and what doesn't count. The cases we suggest here are borderline, related, invented, and contrary cases. Again, these cases may be real-life examples, may come from the literature, or may be constructed by you as exemplars.

Borderline cases are those examples or instances that contain most of the defining attributes of the concept being examined but not all of them. They may contain most or even all of the defining characteristics but differ substantially in one of them, such as length of time or intensity of occurrence. These cases are inconsistent in some way from the concept under consideration, and as such they help us see why the model case is not inconsistent. In this way we help clarify our thinking about the defining attributes of the concept of interest. Again using the coping example, a borderline case might be that of a college student who was facing a big exam. He had not studied until the evening before the test, when he "crammed all night." He finished the examination, but failed the test because he kept falling asleep during the exam. This meets the attributes of covering and protection. However, the example breaks down when it comes to rebalancing. Even though he took the test and may even have known the answers, his continual falling asleep caused him to fail the test. If he were completely rebalanced, thus staying awake, he would probably have passed the test.

Consider the two concepts of anxiety and fear as borderline cases of each other. These two concepts are very closely related to one another and yet are not exactly the same. What makes them different? According to Bay and Algase (1999, p. 107), anxiety is a "heightened sense of uneasiness to a potential threat, which is inconsistent with the expected event and results when there is a mismatch between the next likely event and the actual event." Fear, on the other hand, is a "sufficiently potent, biologically driven, motivated state wherein a single salient threat guides behavior. Fear is a defensive response to perceived threat or the result of exposure to a single cue presented in an environment reminiscent of the original fear experience" (p. 107). Here is a real-life model case of anxiety: A woman is walking in the jungle. She worries that there might be wild animals somewhere around but she doesn't see any or hear any. The model case for fear might be as follows: A woman is walking in the jungle. She worries that there are wild animals around and she hears a lion roaring somewhere. She turns a corner and there is a lion in her path facing her. The primary difference between the two concepts is that fear has a real source of threat to survival, whereas anxiety has an unspecified source of threat. This example shows how distinguishing between the concept under analysis and a concept that is very much like it is crucial to concept development.

Another example of a borderline case may make things even clearer. Because concepts help us classify things, we gave students an exercise in class. We asked them to categorize the contents of their closet. One student classified her clothes as "things I wear above my waist" and "things I wear below my waist." She was puzzled as to how to classify the belts because they were worn *at* the waist. This is a classic, indeed a concrete, example of a borderline case because the belt may fit into either category and yet belongs to neither.

Related cases are instances of concepts that are related to the concept being studied but that do not contain all the defining attributes. They are similar to the concept being studied; they are in some way connected to the main concept. The related cases help us understand how the concept being studied fits into the network of concepts surrounding it. Concepts that could be developed into related cases in our coping example, for instance, might be stress, conflict, achievement, and adaptation.

Related cases are those cases that demonstrate ideas that are very similar to the main concept but that differ from them when examined closely. It is the close examination that helps you clarify what counts as the defining attributes of the concept under analysis and what doesn't count. Related cases have names of their own and should be identified with their names in the analysis. This will help readers see how you made the decisions that you made. It will also help readers determine what the constellation of surrounding concepts looks like.

Haas's (1999a, 1999b) study of quality of life is an excellent example of using related cases to help clarify the defining attributes of the concept. Haas reviewed the literature and found several concepts that were often used interchangeably with quality of life: functional status, satisfaction with life, well-being, and health status. Her careful analysis of how each concept differed from quality of life, substantially aided her in identifying the most robust defining attributes for quality of life.

Contrary cases are clear examples of "not the concept." Again, Wilson (1963) suggests that it can be said of the contrary case, "Well, whatever the concept is, that is certainly not an instance of it." In our coping example, for instance, the contrary case might describe a host who is preparing dinner for a group of people. The roast burns on one end. The host becomes upset, throws out the whole roast, and sends the guests home unfed. We can see from this example the host's behavior is not an example of coping. It meets none of the three critical attributes we have said must pertain to an instance of coping—covering, protection, and rebalancing.

Kissinger's (1998) analysis of the concept of overconfidence has a wonderful example of a contrary case. In the contrary case a nurse finds her patient short of breath, rushes out to another nurse, and says; "What should I do? I've seen her like this before, but I am just so unsure. Please help!" (p. 24). It is clear that whatever overconfidence is, this is not an example of it.

Henson's (1997) study of mutuality is a good example of how negative or contrary cases can help determine the final set of defining attributes. Henson used cases describing paternalism, intrusiveness, and autonomy to help clarify what mutuality was and was not. Henson determined that mutuality actually resided between paternalism and autonomy. It is the middle ground of shared decision making between the obtrusiveness of paternalism on the part of health professionals and the fierce independence of absolute autonomy of the client.

Contrary cases are often very helpful to the analyst because it is often easier to say what something is *not* than what it is. Discovering what a concept is not helps us see in what ways the concept being analyzed is different from the contrary case. This, in turn, gives us information about what the concept should have as defining attributes if the ones from the contrary case are clearly excluded.

Invented cases are cases that contain ideas outside our own experience. They often read like science fiction. Invented cases are useful when you are examining a very familiar concept such as "man," or "love," or one that is so commonplace as to be taken for granted, such as "air." Often to get a true picture of the critical defining attributes, you must take the concept out of its ordinary context and put it into an invented one. Not all concept analyses need invented cases. If the concept is clear and the model case and other cases help you complete the analysis without difficulty or ambiguity, then you probably don't need to use an invented case. They are fun to do, though!

Here is an example using our coping concept. Suppose that a being from another planet visited Earth. Her physiology is such that when she becomes upset or frightened in our atmosphere, she floats straight up into the air, often bumping her head sharply on ceilings. She begins carrying a cement block in her backpack to keep her on the ground. In addition, she pads her helmet and wears it constantly. This is an example of coping in an invented case.

The last type of case is also not always included in a concept analysis. It is the **illegitimate** case. These cases give an example of the concept term used improperly or out of context. In the case of the coping saw, the use of the term *coping* demonstrates neither the attribute of "covering" nor the one of "protection" and so is illegitimately used. These cases are helpful when you come across one meaning for a term that is completely different from all the others. It may have one or two of the critical attributes, but most of the attributes will not apply at all. In the "attachment" analysis at the end of this chapter, the term *attachment* as used to mean those pieces that fit onto a sewing machine contains only the attribute of "touch" and none of the other four.

Once the cases have been put together, they must be compared to the defining attributes one more time to ensure that all the defining attributes have been discovered. Sometimes, once the model case is in place and compared with the other cases and the proposed defining attributes, some areas of overlap, vagueness, or contradiction will become apparent. It is at this point that further refinement becomes necessary. An analysis is not complete until there are no overlapping attributes and no contradictions between the defining attributes and the model case.

Identify Antecedents and Consequences

Identifying antecedents and consequences are the next steps in a concept analysis. Although these two steps are often ignored or dealt with lightly, they may shed considerable light on the social contexts in which the concept is generally used. They are also helpful in further refining the defining attributes. *A defining attribute cannot be either an antecedent or a consequence.* **Antecedents** are those events or incidents that must occur prior to the occurrence of the concept. Thus an antecedent cannot also be a defining attribute for the same concept. For example, Ward (1986) gives a clear example of antecedents of role strain, identifying as the antecedents role conflict, role accumulation, rigidity of time and place, which role demands must be met, and the amount of activity prescribed by some roles. Clearly these antecedents are not the same as role strain itself but must be present for role strain to happen.

Consequences, on the other hand, are those events or incidents that occur as a result of the occurrence of the concept—in other words, the outcomes of the concept. For example, Meraviglia (1999) examined the concept of spirituality and found 12 outcomes resulting from the concept of spirituality. The outcomes were, for example, meaning in life, hope, self-transcendence, trust, creativity, religiousness, and health.

In our coping example, one antecedent was an intensely stressful stimulus (the burned roast); the consequence was the regaining of balance. Another clear example presents itself: If we examine the concept of "pregnancy," one of the antecedents is clearly ovulation, whereas a consequence is some kind of delivery experience whether or not the pregnancy goes to term or produces a viable baby.

In a classic book, Zetterberg (1965) has spoken of constructing theoretical models of determinants and results around a focal variable or construct. (See Chapter 9 for a more thorough discussion of his ideas.) His notion of determinants and results is very close to the notion of antecedents and consequences in concept analysis. Thus, determining antecedents and consequences can be extremely useful theoretically. Antecedents are particularly useful in helping the theorist identify underlying assumptions about the concept being studied. In our attachment example at the end of this chapter, you will see that one of the antecedents is the ability to distinguish between internal and external stimuli. This implies that an assumption of living, sentient beings has been made. Consequences are useful in determining often-neglected ideas, variables, or relationships that may yield fruitful new research directions.

Define Empirical Referents

Determining the empirical referents for the defining attributes is the final step in a concept analysis. When a concept analysis is nearing completion, the question arises, "If we are to measure this concept or determine its existence in the real world, how do we do so?" **Empirical referents** are classes or categories of actual phenomena that by their existence or presence demonstrate the occurrence of the concept itself. As an example, "kissing" might be used as an empirical referent for the concept of "affection." In our coping example an empirical referent might be "ability to successfully solve a problem in a stressful situation." In many cases the defining attributes and the empirical referents will be identical. However, there are times when the concept being analyzed is highly abstract and so are its defining attributes. When that happens, empirical referents are necessary.

Empirical referents, once identified, are extremely useful in instrument development because they are clearly linked to the theoretical base of the concept, thus contributing to both the content and construct validity of any new instrument.

They are also very useful in practice because they provide the clinician with clear, observable phenomena by which to determine the existence of the concept in particular clients. The Boyd (1985), Rew (1986), Meize-Grochowski (1984), and Ward (1986) articles listed in the reference section of this chapter all have good examples of empirical referents.

ADVANTAGES AND LIMITATIONS

Concept analysis clarifies the symbols (words or terms) used in communication. The main advantage of concept analysis is that it renders very precise theoretical as well as operational definitions for use in theory and research. Another advantage is that concept analysis could help clarify those terms in nursing that have become catchphrases and hence have lost their meanings. A third advantage is its utility for tool development and nursing language development. Additionally, the rigorousness of this intellectual exercise is extremely good practice in thinking.

There are few firm rules for concept analysis. Table 5–1 provides several examples of concept analyses using different sets of rules. On the other hand, the theorist must work painstakingly and is likely to encounter pitfalls that will hinder the analysis. These pitfalls, which tend to obscure the meanings you want to convey (Wilson, 1963), include the following:

1. *The tendency to moralize when the concept being analyzed has some value implications.* Many concepts hold some implicit if not explicit value to us. As we begin a concept analysis it is important to recognize that just choosing the concept demonstrates a bias on our part. We must be doubly careful, then, to treat the concept objectively as subject matter rather than subjectively as a persuasive weapon.
2. *The feeling of being absolutely in over your head.* Because there are no firm rules in concept analysis, this may make you very anxious. There is no way we can say to you, "First do this, then do that, and when you have done so, all will be wonderful." We have attempted to give you guidelines, but the actual intellectual work must be yours. Once you have begun, the anxiety subsides and the fun begins.
3. *The feeling that concept analysis is too easy.* Some people initially grow impatient with the process and tend to throw up their hands with the comment, "Well, everybody knows that term means so-and-so. Why do we need to keep on with this?" The point is that not everybody knows what it means. Concept analysis is not easy; it is a vigorous intellectual exercise, but it is fruitful and useful and even enjoyable.
4. *The compulsion to analyze everything, or the "how-do-you-turn-it-off syndrome,"* as one of our students calls it. This occurs fairly often in students. The process of analysis somehow gets their creative juices flowing and they get very excited. The result is often that they don't want to stop. There are some concepts more worthy of analysis than others, but all analyses must finally come to an end. In addition, analysis is only one strategy in theory development. Some energy should be saved for the rest!

TABLE 5–1   EXAMPLES OF CONCEPT ANALYSES

Concept(s)	Author(s)	Journal	Year
Aggregate	Schultz	Adv Nurs Sci	1987
Meaning in suffering	Steeves & Kahn	Image	1987
Health	Simmons	Int J Nurs Stud	1989
Reassurance	Teasdale	J Adv Nurs	1989
Feeling	Beyea	Nurs Diagn	1990
Family management style	Knafl & Deatrick	J Ped Nurs	1990
Quality of life	Oleson	Image	1990
Quality of life	Meeberg	J Adv Nurs	1993
Therapeutic reciprocity	Marck	Adv Nurs Sci	1990
Comfort	Kolcaba	Image	1991
Serenity	Roberts & Fitzgerald	Scholar Inquiry Nurs Pract	1991
Chronic sorrow	Teel	J Adv Nurs	1991
Experience	Watson	J Adv Nurs	1991
Hypothermia	Summers	Nurs Diagn	1992
Spiritual perspective, hope, acceptance, self-transcendence	Hasse, Britt, Coward, Leidy, & Penn	Image	1992
Empathy	Morse, Anderson, Bottorff, Yonge, O'Brien, Solberg, et al.	Image	1992
Pain management	Davis	Adv Nurs Sci	1992
Knowing the patient	Jenny & Logan	Image	1992
Preventive health behavior	Kulbok & Baldwin	Adv Nurs Sci	1992
Fear	Whitley	Nurs Diagn	1992
Unpleasant symptoms	Lenz, Suppe, Gift, Pugh, & Milligan	Adv Nurs Sci	1995
Mutuality	Henson	Image	1997
Unpleasant symptoms	Lenz, Pugh, Milligan, Gift, & Suppe	Adv Nurs Sci	1997
Empowerment	Ellis-Stoll & Popkess-Vawter	Adv Nurs Sci	1998
Overconfidence	Kissinger	Nurs Forum	1998
Ineffective breathing pattern, ineffective airway clearance, & impaired gas exchange	Carlson-Catalano, Lunney, Paradiso, Bruno, Luise, Martin, et al.	Image	1998
Autonomy	Keenan	J Adv Nurs	1999
Pain	Montes-Sandoval	J Adv Nurs	1999
Personal transformation	Wade	J Adv Nurs	1998
Professional nurse autonomy	Wade	J Adv Nurs	1999
Quality of life	Haas	Image	1999
Spirituality	Meraviglia	J Holistic Nurs	1999
Quality of life	Haas	West J Nurs Res	1999

(continued)

TABLE 5–1   Examples of Concept Analyses (CONTINUED)

Concept(s)	Author(s)	Journal	Year
Nursing presence	Doona, Cahse, & Haggerty	J Holistic Nurs	1999
Fear and anxiety	Bay & Algase	Nurs Diagn	1999
Family caregiving skill	Schumacher, Stewart, Archbold, Dodd, & Dibble	Res Nurs & Health	2000
Control	Croom, Procter, & Le Couteur	J Adv Nurs	2000
Chronic confusion, dementia, & impaired environmental interpretation syndrome	Reid & Dassen	Nurs Diagn	2000
Physical touch	Chang	J Adv Nurs	2001
Caregiver abuse	Ayres & Woodtli	J Adv Nurs	2001
Malnutrition in the elderly	Chen, Schilling, & Lyder	J Adv Nurs	2001
Near death experience	Simpson	J Adv Nurs	2001
Equity	Almond	J Adv Nurs	2002
Infant feeding responsiveness	Mentro, Steward, & Garvin	J Adv Nurs	2002
Nursing productivity	Holcomb, Hoffart, & Fox	J Adv Nurs	2002
Self-management	Schilling, Grey, & Knafl	J Adv Nurs	2002
Uncertainty in illness	McCormick	J Nurs Schol	2002

5. *The need to protect oneself from others' criticism or debate* during the process of analysis. Good concept analysis cannot occur in a vacuum. Only the insights and criticisms of others can fully expand the analyst's ideas. The willingness to look foolish is one of the criteria for creativity. If you restrain yourself in discussions or fail to seek criticism because you may look "silly" or "dumb," you are cutting yourself off from successful concept development. In dealing with concept analysis, it is vital to say something and then trust that it will lead somewhere.

6. *The feeling that verbal facility equals thinking.* There is sometimes a tendency to engage in superficial fluency instead of productive dialogue. Most of us know people who can talk or write easily but have little of real substance to say. There are times in concept analysis when the analyst must struggle with difficult and substantive problems. It is often tempting to go for the hasty solution or to beg the question by substituting verbiage for substance. But the results of hasty analysis are meager and unproductive. It is far more helpful to "hang in there" with the difficulties until you solve them in a way that provides the best results, not the easiest.

7. *The attempt to add superfluous defining attributes.* Doing so can confound the results of the analysis because many of the added attributes are not critical to the concept and may even overlap the antecedents and consequences. A rule of thumb is to "quit when you're done" with the original analysis.

Although any or all of these pitfalls may potentially hinder analysis, a sense of proportion, a little risk taking, a sense of humor, and a low anxiety level are all helpful in the process of analysis. This is a new way of thinking for many people and as such requires a little getting used to in the beginning. It is a very important aspect to theory construction. Because concepts are the bricks of theory development, it is critical that they be structurally sound. If a theory contains careful concept analyses, all who read the theory or use it in practice will be able to clearly understand what is meant by the concepts within it and their relationships to each other.

Even beautifully analyzed concepts can contribute merely the basics of theory. Only when concepts are studied for relationships among them and relational statements are constructed can real forward progress be made in theory construction.

UTILIZING THE RESULTS OF CONCEPT ANALYSIS

Several uses of the results of concept analysis have been discussed. These are refining ambiguous terms in theory, education, research, and practice; providing operational definitions with a clear theoretical base; providing an understanding of the underlying attributes of a concept; facilitating instrument development in research; and providing assistance in the development of nursing language.

Once a concept has been analyzed, what is the next step for the theorist? This depends in part on the aims of the analysis. If one of the aims, for instance, is to develop an instrument, then the next step would be to construct items that would reflect the defining attributes of the concept. If the aim is to propose a nursing diagnosis, intervention, or outcome name, then the next step would be to clinically validate the defining attributes. Using the empirical referents for the defining attributes and assessing clients for the presence or absence of the attributes would help substantiate the potential diagnosis, intervention activities, or outcome criteria. If the aim is to construct an operational definition, the next step would be to attempt to find a research instrument that accurately reflects the defining attributes of the concept.

Concept analysis alone will not provide useful theories for nursing education, research, or practice. Only when the concepts are linked to each other will useful theories result (see Chapter 2). In the meantime, scientists, educators, and clinicians should continue to examine concepts critically in an effort to refine nursing knowledge and to discover what those linkages are.

SUMMARY

The process of concept analysis has been the focus of this chapter. This strategy employs the processes of analysis to extract the defining attributes of a concept. There are no rules for accomplishing the analysis. Selection of the concept and the theorist's familiarity with the literature will have some impact on where the theorist begins. The steps in concept analysis include selecting the concept, determining the aims of analysis, identifying all uses of the concept, determining the defining attributes of the concept, identifying model cases, examining additional cases, identifying antecedents and consequences, and determining empirical referents.

Concept analysis increases the richness of our vocabulary and provides precise and rigorously constructed theoretical and operational definitions for use in theory and research. However, concept analysis is limited by the level of theory that can be attained using only concepts. In the next section of this book, we will describe some strategies for going beyond concepts to develop statements about how concepts are related to each other.

Criticism of the method we propose here has implied that the strategy of concept analysis is positivistic, reductionistic, rigid, and requires a correspondence theory of truth (Gift, 1995; Hupcey, Morse, Lenz, & Tasón, 1996; Rodgers, 1989). It has never been our intent to subscribe to these tenets. Indeed, it is not the intent of most current philosophers of science to subscribe to such outmoded views (Schumacher & Gortner, 1992). We have never suggested that our method or Wilson's is the only method of concept analysis. However, concept analysis, using whatever technique, is a reasonable and logical method that has served the development of science in many disciplines over time.

Nursing science will be judged by whether it solves "significant disciplinary problems" (DeGroot, 1988), "offers defensible interpretations of multiple realities of interest to nurses" (Coward, 1990), or provides practitioners with an adequate and holistic knowledge base from which to practice (Avant, 1991). It is our belief that concept analysis, using the method proposed here, will be a useful tool in fulfilling these criteria. We leave it up to the reader to make the final judgment as to the usefulness and validity of the method.

AN ADDITIONAL EXAMPLE AND PRACTICE EXERCISE

To aid you with the subsequent practice exercise, we present below a brief summary of a concept analysis of "attachment." This is by no means a complete, formal analysis. It is presented merely to show how one looks as it is developed.

Concept: Attachment.

Aim of Analysis: Develop operational definition of theoretical concept.

Defining Attributes:

All cases of attachment:

1. Visual contact must have been made between the person and the object of attachment.
2. The person must have touched the object of attachment at some time during the process of attachment.
3. There must be some positive affect associated with the object of attachment.

Cases of animate attachment have the following attributes in addition to the ones above:

4. There must be reciprocal interaction between the two parties in attachment.
5. Vocalization by at least one of the two parties is supportive of attachment process.

Model Cases

Person-to-Object Attachment

A woman explains to her friend that she simply can't throw out her old bathrobe because she has had it since she married and is just too "attached to it."

Person-to-Person Attachment

An 8-month-old boy is playing in the room where his mother is sewing. As he plays, he occasionally looks around at her, or comes over and touches her. When she leaves the room, he cries and begins to search for her. When she returns, he climbs into her lap. She hugs him close and talks to him until he is ready to continue playing.

Contrary Case: Nonattachment

A 22-year-old woman delivers a baby under general anesthesia and cesarean section as a result of abruptio placenta. The infant is about 26 weeks' gestation and weighs 2 pounds. He is immediately transferred to the regional perinatal center 200 miles away. When the mother wakes from anesthesia, she is told she has a 2-pound baby boy and also about his transfer. She is told the baby will stay in the hospital until he weighs about 5 pounds. Due to postpartum complications, the mother is not released from the hospital for 3 weeks. Even though her husband brings reports of the baby, she says, "Do I really have a baby?"

Borderline Case: At-Risk Attachment

Jeffrey is being seen at the health clinic for possible child abuse. Jeffrey is blind due to retrolental fibroplasia. He also has spastic cerebral palsy. Jeffrey's mother says she gets angry because he won't look at her or cuddle when she picks him up. When he cries too long, she hits him. This is borderline attachment because two defining characteristics, touch and vocalization, are met. Visual contact, positive affect, and reciprocal interaction are absent or severely diminished. Attachment may still occur, but it will be difficult.

Related Cases

Love	Deprivation
Separation	Dependency
Detachment	Symbiosis

Illegitimate Case

A salesperson demonstrating a new sewing machine makes a point of explaining "the most useful attachment—the buttonholer."

Antecedents

1. Ability to distinguish between internal and external stimuli.
2. Ability to receive and respond to cues of the persons involved in attachment process.

Consequences

1. Proximity-maintaining behavior
2. Separation anxiety

Empirical Referents—Examples

1. Eye-to-eye contact
2. Patting, stroking, holding hands, etc.
3. Speaking positively about the person
4. Speaking, singing, reading to the person

PRACTICE EXERCISE

Analyze the concept of "play" using the foregoing analysis as a guide. Some of your defining attributes probably were similar to the ones below.

1. Movement or activity
2. One animate entity
3. Voluntariness or choice
4. Expectation of diversion or pleasure
5. Novelty or unpredictability
6. Creativity

Did you remember to include the ideas "play on words," "play in the steering wheel," "play" as in a drama, and so forth?

Using the defining attributes above, develop a model case that includes all of them.

What are some related concepts? How about "games," "work," "exercise," "performance," "imitate," "sport"?

Try developing a contrary case using "work" as "not play." Use the concept "exercise" as a borderline case.

Complete the analysis using the outline given.

REFERENCES

Almond P. An analysis of the concept of equity and its application to health visiting. *J Adv Nurs*. 2002;37(6):598-606.

Avant K. Nursing diagnosis: maternal attachment. *Adv Nurs Sci*. 1979;2(1):45-56.

Avant KC. The theory-research dialectic: a different approach. *Nurs Sci Q*. 1991;4(1):2.

Ayres MM, Woodtli A. Concept analysis: abuse of ageing caregivers by elderly care recipients. *J Adv Nurs*. 2001;35(3):326-334.

Bay EJ, Algase DL. Fear and anxiety: a simultaneous concept analysis. *Nurs Diagn*. 1999;10(3):103-111.

Beyea SC. Concept analysis of feeling: a human response pattern. *Nurs Diagn*. 1990;1(3):97-101.

Boyd C. Toward an understanding of mother–daughter identification using concept analysis. *Adv Nurs Sci*. 1985;7(3):78-86.

Carlson-Catalano J, Lunney M, Paradiso C, Bruno J, Luise BK, Martin T, et al. Clinical validation of ineffective breathing pattern, ineffective airway clearance, and impaired gas exchange. *Image*. 1998;30(3):243-248.

Chang SO. The conceptual structure of physical touch in caring. *J Adv Nurs*. 2001;33(6):820-827.

Chase S. Response to "The concept of nursing presence: state of the science." *Scholar Inquiry Nurs Pract*. 2001;15(4):323-325.

Chen CCH, Schilling LS, Lyder CH. A concept analysis of malnutrition in the elderly. *J Adv Nurs*. 2001;36(1):131-142.

Coward DD. Critical multiplism: a research strategy for nursing science. *Image*. 1990;22(3):163-166.

Croom S, Procter S, Le Couteur A. Developing a concept analysis of control for use in child and adolescent mental health nursing. *J Adv Nurs*. 2000;31(6):1324-1332.

Davis G. The meaning of pain management: a concept analysis. *Adv Nurs Sci*. 1992;15(1):77-86.

DeGroot HA. Scientific inquiry in nursing: a model for a new age. *Adv Nurs Sci*. 1988;10(3):1-21.

Doona ME, Chase SK, Haggerty LA. Nursing presence: as real as a Milky Way bar. *J Holistic Nurs*. 1999;17(1):54-70.

Ellis-Stoll CC, Popkess-Vawter S. A concept analysis on the process of empowerment. *Adv Nurs Sci*. 1998;21(2):62-68.

Gamel C, Grypdonck M, Hengveld M, Davis B. A method to develop a nursing intervention: the contribution of qualitative studies to the process. *J Adv Nurs*. 2001;33(6):806-819.

Gift AG, ed. Concept development in nursing. *Scholar Inquiry Nurs Pract*. 1995;10(3, special issue).

Gordon M. *Nursing Diagnosis: Process and Application*. New York, NY: McGraw-Hill; 1982.

Haas BK. A multidisciplinary concept analysis of quality of life. *West J Nurs Res*. 1999a;21(6):728-742.

Haas BK. Clarification and integration of similar quality of life concepts. *Image*. 1999b;31(3):215-220.

Haase JE, Britt T, Coward DD, Leidy NK, Penn PE. Simultaneous concept analysis of spiritual perspective, hope, acceptance, and self-transcendence. *Image*. 1992;24(2):141-147.

Henson RH. Analysis of the concept of mutuality. *Image*.1997;29(1):77-81.

Holcomb BR, Hoffart N, Fox MH. Defining and measuring nursing productivity: a concept analysis and pilot study. *J Adv Nurs*. 2002;38(4): 378-386.

Hupcey JE, Morse JM, Lenz ER, Tasón M. Wilsonian methods of concept analysis: a critique. *Scholar Inquiry Nurs Pract*. 1996;10(3):185-210.

Jenny J, Logan J. Knowing the patient: one aspect of clinical knowledge. *Image*. 1992;24(4):254-258.

Keenan J. A concept analysis of autonomy. *J Adv Nurs*. 1999;29(3):556-562.

Kissinger JA. Overconfidence: a concept analysis. *Nurs Forum*. 1998;33(2):18-26.

Knafl KA, Deatrick JA. Family management style: concept analysis and development. *J Pediatr Nurs*. 1990;5(1):4-14.

Kolcaba KY. A taxonomic structure for the concept comfort. *Image*. 1991;23(4):237-240.

Kulbok PA, Baldwin JH. From preventive health behavior to health promotion: advancing a positive construct of health. *Adv Nurs Sci*. 1992;14(4):50-64.

Lenz, ER, Pugh LC, Milligan RA, Gift A, Suppe F. The middle-range theory of unpleasant symptoms. *Adv Nurs Sci*. 1997;19(3):14-27.

Lenz ER, Suppe F, Gift AG, Pugh LC, Milligan RA. Collaborative development of middle-range nursing theories: toward a theory of unpleasant symptoms. *Adv Nurs Sci.* 1995;17(3):1-13.

Marck P. Therapeutic reciprocity: a caring phenomenon. *Adv Nurs Sci.* 1990;13(1):49-59.

McCormick KM. A concept analysis of uncertainty in illness. *J Nurs Schol.* 2002;34(2):127-131.

Meeberg GA. Quality of life: a concept analysis. *J Adv Nurs.* 1993;18:32-38.

Meize-Grochowski R. An analysis of the concept of trust. *J Adv Nurs.* 1984;9:563-572.

Mentro AM, Steward DK, Garvin BJ. Infant feeding responsiveness: a conceptual analysis. *J Adv Nurs.* 2002;37(2):208-216.

Meraviglia MG. Critical analysis of spirituality and its empirical indicators: prayer and meaning in life. *J Holistic Nurs.* 1999;17(1):18-33.

Montes-Sandoval L. An analysis of the concept of pain. *J Adv Nurs.* 1999;29(4):935-941.

Morse JM, Anderson G, Bottorff JL, Yonge O, O'Brien B, Solberg SM, et al. Exploring empathy: a conceptual fit for nursing practice. *Image.* 1992;24(4):273-280.

Nunnally J. *Psychometric Theory.* New York, NY: McGraw-Hill; 1978.

Oleson M. Subjectively perceived quality of life. *Image.* 1990;22(3):187-190.

Reid S, Dassen T. Chronic confusion, dementia, and impaired environmental interpretation syndrome: a concept comparison. *Nurs Diagn.* 2000;11(2):49-59.

Rew L. Intuition: concept analysis of a group phenomenon. *Adv Nurs Sci.* 1986; 8(2):21-28.

Reynolds PD. *A Primer in Theory Construction.* Indianapolis, Ind: Bobbs-Merrill; 1971.

Roberts KT, Fitzgerald L. Serenity: caring with perspective. *Scholar Inquiry Nurs Pract.* 1991;5(2):127-141.

Rodgers BL. Concepts, analysis and the development of nursing knowledge: the evolutionary cycle. *J Adv Nurs.* 1989;14:330-335.

Schilling LS, Grey M, Knafl KA. The concept of self-management of type 1 diabetes in children and adolescents: an evolutionary concept analysis. *J Adv Nurs.* 2002;37(1):87-99.

Schultz PR. When the client means more than one: extending the foundational concept of person. *Adv Nurs Sci.* 1987;10(1):71-86.

Schumacher KL, Gortner SR. (Mis)conceptions and reconceptions about traditional science. *Adv Nurs Sci.* 1992;14(4):1-11.

Schumacher KL, Stewart BJ, Archbold PG, Dodd MJ, Dibble SL. Family caregiving skill: development of the concept. *Res Nurs Health.* 2000;23:191-203.

Simmons SJ. Health: a concept analysis. *Int J Nurs Stud.* 1989;26(2):155-161.

Simpson SM. Near death experience: a concept analysis as applied to nursing. *J Adv Nurs.* 2001;36(4):520-526.

Smith TD. The concept of nursing presence: state of the science. *Scholar Inquiry Nurs Pract.* 2001;15(4):299-322.

Steeves RH, Kahn DL. Experience of meaning in suffering. *Image.* 1987;19(3):114-116.

Summers S. Hypothermia: one nursing diagnosis or three? *Nurs Diagn.*1992;3(1):2-11.

Teasdale K. The concept of reassurance in nursing. *J Adv Nurs.* 1989;14:444-450.

Teel CS. Chronic sorrow: analysis of the concept. *J Adv Nurs.* 1991;16:1311-1319.

Wade GH. A concept analysis of personal transformation. *J Adv Nurs.* 1998;28(4):713-719.

Wade GH. Professional nurse autonomy: concept analysis and application to nursing education. *J Adv Nurs.* 1999;30(2):310-318.

Ward C. The meaning of role strain. *Adv Nurs Sci.* 1986;8(2):39-49.

Watson SJ. An analysis of the concept of experience. *J Adv Nurs.* 1991;16:1117-1121.

Whitley GG. Concept analysis as foundational to nursing diagnosis research. *Nurs Diagn.* 1995;6(2):91-92.

Whitley GG. Concept analysis of fear. *Nurs Diagn.* 1992;3(4):155-161.

Wilson J. *Thinking with Concepts.* New York, NY: Cambridge University Press; 1963.

Zetterberg HL. *On theory and verification in sociology.* Totowa, NJ: Bedminster Press, 1965.

ADDITIONAL READINGS

Arakelian M. An assessment and nursing application of the concept of locus of control. *Adv Nurs Sci.* 1980;3(1):25-42.

Brown AJ. A concept analysis of respect: applying the hybrid model in cross-cultural settings. *West J Nurs Res.* 1997;19(6):762-780.

Carnevali D. Conceptualizing, a nursing skill. In: Mitchell PH, ed. *Concepts Basic to Nursing.* 2nd ed. New York, NY: McGraw-Hill; 1977.

Carper B. Fundamental patterns of knowing in nursing. *Adv Nurs Sci.* 1978;1(1):13-23.

Chinn PL, Jacobs K. A model for theory development in nursing. *Adv Nurs Sci.* 1978;1(1):1-12.

Deatrick JA, Knafl KA, Murphy-Moore C. Clarifying the concept of normalization. *Image.* 1999;31(3):209-214.

Doona ME, Haggerty LA, Chase SK. Nursing presence: an existential exploration of the concept. *Scholar Inquiry Nurs Pract.* 1997;11(1):3-20.

Englemann S. *Conceptual Learning.* San Rafael, Calif: Dimensions; 1969.

Goulet C, Bell L, Tribble DS, Paul D, Lang A. A concept analysis of parent-infant attachment. *J Adv Nurs.* 1998;28(5):1071-1081.

Hempel CG. *Fundamentals of Concept Formation in Empirical Science.* Chicago, Ill: University of Chicago Press; 1952.

Hupcey JE, Penrod J, Morse JM, Mitcham C. An exploration and advancement of the concept of trust. *J Adv Nurs.* 2001;36(2):282-293.

Hutchfield K. Family-centred care: a concept analysis. *J Adv Nurs.* 1999;29(5):1178-1187.

Jenner CA. The art of nursing: a concept analysis. *Nurs Forum.* 1997;32(4):5-11.

Klausmeier HJ, Ripple RE. *Learning and Human Abilities.* New York, NY: Harper & Row; 1971.

Kunyk D, Olson JK. Clarification of conceptualizations of empathy. *J Adv Nurs.* 2001; 35(3):317-325.

Lyth GM. Clinical supervision: a concept analysis. *J Adv Nurs.* 2000;31(3):722-729.

Maijala H, Munnukka T, Nikkonen M. Feeling of "lacking" as the core of envy: a conceptual analysis of envy. *J Adv Nurs.* 2000;31(6):1342-1350.

Matthews C, Gaul A. Nursing diagnosis from the perspective of concept attainment and critical thinking. *Adv Nurs Sci.* 1979;2(1):17-26.

Norris CM. Restlessness: a nursing phenomenon in search of meaning. *Nurs Outlook.* 1975; 23:103-107.

Paley J. Positivism and qualitative nursing research. *Scholar Inquiry Nurs Pract.* 2001;15(4):371-387.

Penrod J. Refinement of the concept of uncertainty. *J Adv Nurs.* 2001;34(2):238-245.

Popper KR. *Conjectures and Refutations.* 4th ed. London, England: Rutledge & Kegan Paul; 1972.

Rawnsley M. The concept of privacy. *Adv Nurs Sci.* 1980;2(2):25-32.

Richmond JP, McKenna H. Homophobia: an evolutionary analysis of the concept as applied to nursing. *J Adv Nurs.* 1998;28(2):362-369.

Roberts KT, Whall A. Serenity as a goal for nursing practice. *Image.* 1996;28(4):359-364.

Robinson DS, McKenna HP. Loss: an analysis of a concept of particular interest to nursing. *J Adv Nurs.* 1998;27:779-784.

Rodgers BL, Kanfl KA. *Concept Development in Nursing: Foundations, Techniques, and Applications.* 2nd ed. Philadelphia, Penn: WB Saunders; 1999.

Ryles SM. A concept analysis of empowerment: its relationship to mental health nursing. *J Adv Nurs.* 1999;29(3):600-607.

Smith J. The idea of health: a philosophical inquiry. *Adv Nurs Sci.* 1981;3(3):43-50.

Schoenfelder DP, Crowell CM, and the NDEC Team. From risk for trauma to unintentional injury risk: falls—a concept analysis. *Nurs Diagn.* 1999;10(4):149-157.

Stern PN. Grounded theory methodology: its uses and processes. *Image.* 1980;12(2):20-23.

Suppe F. Response to "positivism and qualitative nursing research." *Scholar Inquiry Nurs Pract.* 2001;15(4):389-397.

Swanson EA, Hensen DP, Specht J, Johnson ML, Maas M. Caregiving: concept analysis and outcomes. *Scholar Inquiry Nurs Pract.* 1997;11(1):65-79.

Wall LM. Exercise: a unitary concept. *Nurs Sci Q.* 1999;12(1):68-72.

PART III

Statement Development

Developing statements is an important aspect of theory development. Laws and empirical generalizations, both being forms of scientific statements, supply much of the working backbone of science. In a practice discipline, many of the diagnoses, interventions, or outcomes of practice may be based on such scientific statements. For example, Yeh (2002) hypothesized that there would be gender differences in the levels of stress and psychological distress experienced by parents whose children had cancer. Mothers in her study showed significantly higher scores on both stress and distress than did fathers. Yeh suggests that appropriate counseling and other interventions may be different for fathers and mothers. Thus, for practice, statement development can be a very important and useful level of theory development. It is especially relevant when a theorist wishes to go beyond the concept (naming) phase but does not need the comprehensive perspectives offered by a theory.

Selecting the statement development strategy most suitable to a theorist's purposes involves assessing the "state of the art" of existing knowledge about one's topic of interest. To make this assessment, first clearly identify what the topic of interest is. Then read key articles or references that are up to date and capture the main ideas about the topic of interest. If a topic is new, it is likely that available resources will not be very comprehensive. After reading materials carefully, form your judgment about the state of the art.

When assessment of the existing literature shows the topic of interest to be undeveloped, or simply outmoded and in need of a fresh start, statement synthesis (Chapter 6) or statement derivation (Chapter 7) may be appropriate. In the former situation, statement synthesis can be undertaken if the theorist has the resources and inclination for collecting and analyzing observations, either qualitatively or quantitatively; if this is not so, statement derivation can be undertaken. If the literature primarily contains research findings that need to be integrated, then literary methods of statement synthesis (Chapter 6) may be suitable. Finally, if the literature is well developed but not research based, statement analysis (Chapter 8) may be a useful starting strategy. Although more than one strategy may be suited to the state of a topical area, it is advisable to select one and use it until it ceases to be useful rather than trying to use two or three strategies simultaneously.

REFERENCE

Yeh C. Gender differences of parental distress in children with cancer. *J Adv Nurs.* 2002; 38(6):598-606.

6

Statement Synthesis

Preliminary Note: *If concepts synthesized from practice or research are the building blocks of theory, then theoretical statements are the mortar that glues each block to its neighbor. In developing statements of relationships between concepts, the theory builder starts to bring clarity and direction to the understanding of phenomena of interest. Statement synthesis may contribute to knowledge about simple two-factor relationships. More typically, though, statement synthesis is an incremental phase essential to the larger goal of theory synthesis. Thus, statement synthesis is part of the incremental process of theory development, especially when one moves from observations or data to general statements.*

DEFINITION AND DESCRIPTION

As a strategy, statement synthesis is aimed at specifying relationships between two or more concepts based on evidence. The evidence may come from various sources: (1) qualitative or quantitative methods applied to observations or interviews of individuals or groups; or (2) literature-based sources such as literature reviews, conclusions extracted from interrelated studies, standards of practice, or practice guidelines.

(*Note:* Readers may find it helpful to review the material on the nature of statements in Chapter 2 before proceeding further in this chapter.)

Logically, statement synthesis involves two operations: moving from evidence to inferences, and then generalizing from specific inferences to more abstract ones. In the first of these operations, evidence is comprised of a thoughtful series of observations that are the basis of interrelating concepts. For example, a nurse may interview caregivers of elderly patients in nursing homes about the experience of caring for an elder. From qualitative analysis of the interview transcripts, clusters of related ideas about the social experience of caring for elders are constructed. The nurse then links related clusters into relational statements such as: *Caregivers of elders in nursing homes relate more fully to elders when they have a sense of an elder's life story before coming to the nursing home* (see Figure 6–1a).

A second source of evidence for statement synthesis uses statistical methods to compress many individual observations or measurements. Quantitative indices,

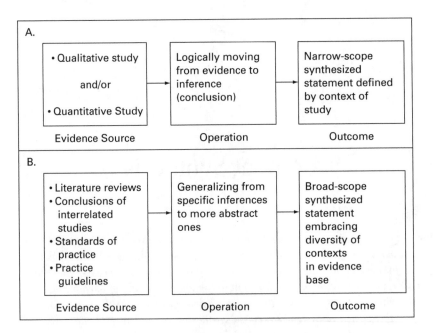

FIGURE 6–1   Evidence-based statement synthesis.

such as correlation coefficients, can describe the presence and strength of a relationship between two variables. In this situation, statement synthesis permits relationships expressed in numerical form to be translated into verbal or linguistic form. For example, suppose a nurse gathers data about two variables, acculturation and emotional eating, and finds the correlation between them as $r = 0.50$, $p <.05$. One way this statistical information could be expressed is: *As acculturation increases, emotional eating increases.* Statistically based statement synthesis can be applied to both descriptive (nonexperimental) research and experimental research studies.

In the third source of evidence, a theorist undertakes statement synthesis about a topic for which much research already exists in published documents (see Figure 6–1b). For example, you might do an electronic search of research literature to locate factors that affect the success of patient education programs and the outcomes that result from patient education. The process of synthesis might begin by cataloging relationships among variables reported in the literature retrieved. Relationships would then be further organized and combined to obtain clear and general statements of relationships among concepts. Because some relationships may be found repeatedly in studies, whereas others may be found in only one or two studies, statements may be grouped according to how much evidence is available for each one. The result of this work would ideally be several statements that capture the broad patterns of relationships among variables that are evident in the literature.

These introductory illustrations of statement synthesis show that this strategy consists of multiple and varied methods. The desired outcome of these diverse methods, however, is the same: the clear statement of relationships between two or more concepts. Furthermore, the theorist using statement synthesis pulls together, organizes, or extracts patterns of relationships from information gathered in reality—the outside world. Thus, observations and other methods of scientific measurement, for example, interviews and machine readings, are essential to the process of statement synthesis. Unlike other statement development strategies, statement synthesis requires empirical evidence in some form as a beginning point.

For interested readers, a *self-assessment test* of introductory statistics is located at the end of this chapter. Obtaining maximum benefit from quantitative methods presented in this chapter may be enhanced by knowledge of introductory statistics. Readers may use this self-assessment to assess or refresh their knowledge of statistics. Several helpful statistical texts also are listed at the end of this chapter for interested readers.

Nevertheless, mastery of statistics is not essential for every method of statement synthesis. Familiarity with statistical methods, however, is an indispensable tool when large amounts of quantitative information are collected. Statistical methods may be useful in consolidating large amounts of collected information into a more interpretable form. Nonetheless, readers should not confuse statistics with statement synthesis. Statistical methods are only adjuncts to the process of specifying relationships among concepts in the field of interest.

PURPOSE AND USES

The purpose of statement synthesis is to develop from observations of phenomena one or more statements about relationships that exist among those phenomena. As indicated earlier, the observations may be made directly by the theorist or may be drawn from the literature. Further, where large numbers of quantitative observations or measurements are made, these may be treated statistically to compress the information into a more interpretable form.

Although data or observations may be used to develop or to test hypotheses, these two uses are quite distinct. However, similar techniques may be employed in each of these two purposes. This similarity leads to several confusions. Theorists may needlessly apply rules for justification to a discovery context (see Chapter 1). For example, statistical results with a probability level slightly greater than .05 might be disregarded needlessly, even though the finding makes sense conceptually in exploratory analyses.

Conversely, theorists may discover certain relationships among phenomena using a loose pragmatic research design but then treat the "discovery" as if it were a well-proven fact. As noted in Chapter 1, it is preferable, as a general rule, to keep the contexts of justification and discovery distinct. Where data are used to extract relational statements (context of discovery), these same data should not be used again to claim the statements have been "tested" (context of justification). As a general rule, another independent data set should be used to confirm or cross-validate the original findings. Similarly, rigorous testing of hypotheses (context of justification) may be followed by further atheoretical analyses or "massaging" of the data (context of discovery). The latter, although important, does not carry the same evidential status as the former type of analysis.

Evidence used for statement synthesis (context of discovery) should be analyzed in ways that facilitate discovery. This may necessitate altering conventions such as traditional probability levels or using exploratory approaches such as bivariate statistical descriptions (Polit, 1996) to construct statements that meaningfully reflect relationships inherent in data or observations. Such flexibility may be wise and appropriate to maximally make use of information collected about a phenomenon in a discovery context. More rigorous approaches would be needed in a justificatory context. For example, improvements in measurement and conceptualization may occur that permit preliminary "discovery" observations to be more suitably and rigorously tested in a later stage of scientific refinement.

When selecting statement synthesis as a strategy for theory construction, theorists should consider that it is especially suited to situations in which one of the following is true: (1) There is no conceptual or empirical work done to describe a topic of interest, but a series of observations can be made readily to establish some of the parameters (empirical qualities) of the phenomenon. (2) There are several concepts in use in an area of interest, but evidence is needed to clarify how the concepts may be interrelated. (3) There are several published research studies on a phenomenon of interest, but the information contained in them has not been organized together or amalgamated.

PROCEDURES FOR STATEMENT SYNTHESIS

Statement synthesis involves two basic logical operations: moving from observations to inferences, and then generalizing from specific inferences to more abstract ones (see Figure 6-1). Two broad classes of methods exist for moving from observations to inferences: qualitative methods and quantitative methods. Generalizing from specific inferences to more general ones, the second operation, is facilitated by a process we have termed literary methods. In actual statement development, a theorist may of course move back and forth between these logical operations.

The complex and voluminous information about qualitative and quantitative methods makes a comprehensive exposition of each beyond the scope of this chapter. Instead, we focus on strategic aspects of these two methods and must necessarily be selective in our presentation of them. Readers needing more in-depth information about qualitative methods are referred to methods texts devoted exclusively to this topic (e.g., Denzin & Lincoln, 2000; Schreiber & Stern, 2001; Strauss & Corbin, 1998). Similarly, for more information about quantitative methods, standard research textbooks are available on this topic (e.g., Pedhazur & Schmelkin, 1991; Polit & Beck, 2003). Keeping these limitations in mind, we present a treatment of qualitative, quantitative, and literary methods as they relate strategically to developing statements about a phenomenon of interest.

Although qualitative methods as a group vary in their purpose and specific method, typically a flexible or modifiable approach is utilized in data collection. This permits the theorist to select observations related to the emerging picture of a phenomenon. Qualitative methods typically rely on interview (listening and questioning) and observation (watching) as sources of data. Coding categories generally emerge from reading and preliminary coding of transcribed interviews supplemented by observational notes. Grounded theory, a qualitative method that may contribute to statement synthesis, is presented below.

In contrast, quantitative methods involve measurement of variables on numerical scales. Quantitative methods may be applied to both experimental and nonexperimental (descriptive or correlational) designs. Quantitative methods may be used to examine relationships between two or more factors, or differing patterns of response to a common event. Translating statistical information into conclusions expressed in linguistic form is a vehicle for statement synthesis.

Last, literary methods are aimed at organizing extant research information on a topic of interest. Sources of evidence in literary methods rely heavily on library and printed materials. Literary methods involve sifting through available information and putting that information into more compact and general form. In some instances the theorist's work of literary statement synthesis will be expedited by the availability of comprehensive literature reviews, well-articulated standards of practice, or practice guidelines on topics of concern.

Qualitative Methods

Grounded theory was one of the early qualitative approaches that lent itself to statement development (Glaser, 1978; Glaser & Strauss, 1967). It was used by nurses to study, for example, patients who underwent mastectomies (Quint, 1967a, 1967b), stepparent families (Stern, 1980), and families across life-cycle stages (Knafl & Grace, 1978). In grounded theory as a method the theorist gains understanding of social phenomena by beginning with an open mind, avoiding preconceived ideas about ways of classifying and interrelating data, and observing social phenomena in natural settings. Although a theorist may begin with some general ideas about the area of interest, these are abandoned as categories more relevant to the phenomenon emerge. The theorist moves back and forth between data collection and data analysis in order to validate emerging ideas and refine concepts and relationships as new data are collected.

The strength of grounded theory is that the theorist uses direct observation of the phenomenon as the starting point for concept and then statement formation (Glaser, 1978; Glaser & Strauss, 1967; Quint, 1967a; Schatzman & Strauss, 1973; Strauss & Corbin, 1998). Data are coded into categories and categories are interrelated as an ongoing part of the data analysis. A theorist may make observations, code them, make interpretive notes or memos about coded observations, and then make further observations to refine or clarify an emerging idea. The theorist's creative ability to construct meaningful general concepts and relational statements is a crucial part of qualitative research. See Benoliel (1996) or Eaves (2001) for a fuller overview of grounded theory methods.

A classic example illustrating grounded theory is Stern's (1980) work with stepfather families. Stern began her study by noting that the process by which a stepfather was integrated into an existing family had not been studied before.

> *I had no basis on which to test existing theory, nor could I utilize identified existing variables, because none were identified. In other words, it was first necessary to find out what was going on in these families. (p. 20)*

In phase one, the *collection of empirical data*, Stern conducted intensive interviews with 30 stepfather families from a variety of social classes and ethnic groups. Data collected by observation and interviews were coded according to their main substance, and similarly coded data were then clustered together in categories. Two categories that Stern developed, for example, focused on rules in the family and enforcement techniques.

During the second phase, *concept formation*, a conceptual framework was developed with an eye to representing the phenomenon from the subjects' point of view. In attempting to understand how families integrate a stepfather into the existing mother–child system, Stern selected the discipline of children in the family as the framework. This framework was selected because of the emotional responses the topic of discipline produced when discussed with families.

The third phase, *concept development*, involved several steps. Categories were linked together to define key variables. Thus, Stern combined the categories of teaching, accepting, and copying into a larger umbrella category of affiliating actions. Common to affiliating actions was bringing the stepfather and child closer together. Emerging ideas necessitated further review of literature at this point. Attention also turned to relationships between categories. In Stern's (1980) study she asked, "under what conditions do the variables discipline and integration coexist?" (p. 22). Data were selectively sampled to clarify the relationship of these variables. Stern found that discipline and integration occurred together only when affiliating actions were also present. This demonstrates statement synthesis. To further consolidate thinking, a core variable was proposed. Core variables pull together key ideas about a phenomenon. Stern proposed "integrative discipline" as the core variable to explain how stepfather families use the issue of discipline to strengthen family solidarity.

During the fourth phase, *concept modification and integration*, the emerging ideas were further integrated and delimited. Data were coded in terms of theoretical ideas. Memos or interpretive notes were made as data were coded to aid in systematizing the findings of the study. Memos were then reorganized in a manner that facilitated the fifth phase, *production of the research report*. In this final phase, theoretical outcomes of the study were presented, substantiated by examples from the data.

Stern's application of grounded theory illustrates a flexible, yet sensitive means of constructing statements about a social phenomenon. This method permits categories and relationships among these to be constructed from direct and thoughtful interaction of the theorist and the social phenomenon being studied. See Benoliel (1996) for a comprehensive listing of nursing studies using grounded theory, 1980–1994.

Quantitative Methods

In this chapter quantitative methods are examined within the framework of experimental and nonexperimental research. In experimental designs, some change is introduced by the investigator to determine its impact on outcomes, whereas in nonexperimental quantitative designs variation is observed as it naturally occurs. Each of these designs for quantitative research involves the collection and analysis of numerical data. The analysis of data typically is facilitated by statistical calculations such as means, standard deviations, percentages, correlation coefficients, and t test and F ratio values. Each of these designs contains some special advantages and limitations for the construction of statements about phenomena. To begin, each design will be described briefly, and then the group nonexperimental design will be presented to illustrate its use in statistically based statement synthesis.

Interpreting statistical data from quantitative-based studies assumes that the measurements used are reliable (Aiken, 1996; Anastasi, 1997; Cronbach, 1997; Nunnally & Bernstein, 1994; Waltz, Strickland, & Lenz, 1991). Validity of measures, particularly construct validity, may be less clear, however, given the reciprocal relationship between theory development and establishment of construct validity (Cronbach & Meehl, 1967). Whereas it is beyond the scope of this chapter to deal with psychometric concepts such as reliability and validity as these affect the interpretation of statistical data, we must acknowledge the presence of these issues to provide a complete and accurate picture of quantitative methods.

Experimental Designs.   These designs are used to document the effects of nursing interventions in diverse situations. For example, Table 6–1 and Figure 6–2

TABLE 6–1 INDIVIDUAL AND MEAN ANXIETY LEVELS FOR PATIENTS PRIOR TO EXPLORATORY SURGERY (FICTITIOUS DATA)

Patient ID	Before Hospitalization	After Admission	After Preoperative Education
Patient A	50	20	20
Patient B	30	40	60
Patient C	30	50	30
Patient D	30	50	30
Group Mean	35	40	35

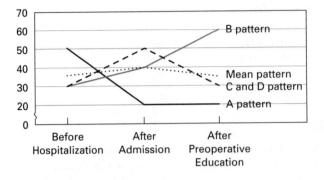

FIGURE 6–2   Individual and mean anxiety levels for patients prior to exploratory surgery (fictitious data).

show fictitious data on four patients having exploratory surgery. A nursing intervention of preoperative education is tested for its impact on reducing patients' anxiety. Mean scores describe the level of anxiety in the group at each time point and estimate the impact of the intervention on reducing anxiety. Examining the group means (bottom row of data) for anxiety level before hospitalization, after admission, and then after preoperative education shows that hospital admission led to an increase in anxiety that was then quelled by preoperative education. For subgroups of individuals, however, the mean gives a misleading estimate of the intervention impact on them.

Looking at individual patients' patterns (top four rows of data), hospital admission appeared to be a relief to Patient A and reduced his anxiety level to well below preadmission levels. For Patient B, admission did raise her anxiety level somewhat, but worse yet, the preoperative education backfired and raised her level of anxiety still higher. Only Patients C and D had individual patterns that generally conformed to those of the group mean. Thus, a second important goal in analyzing data for statement synthesis about nursing interventions is to determine who will benefit from an intervention and who will not. Now, suppose we are able to look at the fictitious patients' data further and learn that Patient A was very worried about some family conflicts that resolved just as he was being admitted to the hospital. He saw the upcoming surgery as a "piece of cake" compared to the difficult family problems. Patient B, however, just had an important support person move out of town as she was being admitted. Patient B felt very fearful about going through the surgery alone and this feeling increased after the preoperative intervention.

In our preoperative education example, patients were tested both before and after the experimental intervention so that change in anxiety could be compared on the same people across time points. In another variation of an experimental design, a control group whose members receive no intervention also may be included so that the effects of the experimental condition may be contrasted with the effects of the control condition. In any circumstances where it would be considered unethical to withhold some form of intervention, the control is converted to a "usual care" group so that there is no question of them receiving needed care. Comparisons made between groups are a way of determining the impact of the intervention in the "experimental" group using the control group as a reference point.

In these various types of experimental studies, statement synthesis occurs as the researcher translates numerical or statistical measures of impact into linguistic form. For our fictitious patients' data, we might develop the following statement:

> *Preoperative education led to a reduction in anxiety for 50% of preoperative patients; interpersonal changes in some patients' lives moderated the effectiveness of the intervention.*

Most readers are already familiar with experimental studies and the type of conclusions that are reached about "main effects." For example: *A support intervention was more successful in reducing depressive symptoms of new immigrants compared to an intervention involving referral to primary care.* We therefore also want to consider findings about differential benefit from an experimental intervention. In an actual example of testing for differential benefit, Kiernan, King, Kraemer, Stefanick, and Killen (1998) examined data from a weight-loss intervention. They used signal detection (involving chi-square tests) to determine what characteristics of participants affected successful weight loss (defined as loss of at least 2 body mass index units). Signal detection methods can aid in partitioning a larger group into successive subgroups who vary in rates of success on the key outcome. First, they found that the nature of the weight-loss program affected success rates, with those in a diet-only group being less successful than those in a diet-and-exercise-class group. Beyond this, Kiernan et al. identified subgroups within the diet-and-exercise-class group who were less or more successful. For example, persons who reported high body image dissatisfaction had difficulty being successful. Among those who were satisfied with their body image, further subgroups were found according to whether or not they had a history of multiple weight-loss attempts. Based on Kiernan and colleagues' work, one statement of differential impact might be expressed as: *Persons with high body image dissatisfaction are less likely to benefit from a weight-loss intervention that includes exercise classes.* This synthesized statement points to the need for new ways to increase exercise in persons with high body image concerns, such as at home-based exercise that does not require exercising in a group context. (*Note:* Our presentation of the work of Kiernan et al. is offered for illustrative purposes. Because the findings reflect only one study, they should not be viewed as definitive.)

Nonexperimental Designs.   These designs often rely on correlation or regression techniques to statistically interrelate variables. Data may be cross-sectional (collected at one time point) or longitudinal (collected over several time points). Although we will not discuss the variety of test statistics that may be used in nonexperimental (also called correlational or *ex post facto*) designs, we will discuss general strategies for the analysis and interpretation of nonexperimental data. Associated statistical and design issues are well treated in available research texts (e.g., Pedhazur & Schmelkin, 1991; Polit & Beck, 2003).

One of the most daunting problems that nonexperimental designs pose for a theorist is the risk of becoming buried in a sea of statistical information. The "shot-gun" approach often used in nonexperimental designs can result in every variable being related to every other variable in the study. In a study of 10 variables (for example, social class, age, gender, number of drugs, number of hospital admissions, etc.), if each of these is correlated with every other variable, a total of 45 correlation coefficients will be generated. In a study of 100 variables, 4,950 variable relationships are possible. Immediately it becomes clear that strategies are needed to eliminate unnecessary statistical analyses and to organize those that are done into meaningful units of information. This is one of the most difficult tasks that faces a theorist using quantitative nonexperimental evidence for statement synthesis.

We recommend several guidelines to aid in organizing the process of data analysis and interpretation:

1. Locate the most focal variables, those of greatest interest to you. Some variables are of interest for their own sake—for example, levels of adjustment or well-being before or after illness. Other variables are of interest only insofar as they may influence focal variables.
2. Examine the statistical indicators of central tendency and variability for the focal variables. If these variables are measured over several occasions, become familiar with changes that may occur in them.
3. Examine related literature for variables that have been found to covary with these focal variables.
4. Determine if your focal variables are related as expected to these variables identified in the literature.
5. Reduce variables that seem to have a common orientation by such procedures as factor analysis (Tabachnick & Fidell, 2001), if possible. Social background variables can often be made more compact by this approach.
6. Follow up hunches that you may have about new variables in your data set that you suspect may be related to the focal variables.
7. Look for "surprises" in the data analysis results. These may be unanticipated relationships or unanticipated lack of relationships. Hypothesize about why these surprises may have occurred. Check out your hypotheses to the extent possible with your available data. These hypotheses, even though moving beyond statement synthesis itself, may be helpful for later theory synthesis.
8. You may have started out atheoretically (without any theory in mind to be proven), but you may find during the data analysis and interpretation phase that the results obtained are consistent with available theories. These theories may in turn suggest new or previously unexplored areas for further analysis.

9. Discuss results obtained with colleagues knowledgeable in the area as well as with clinicians who know the area under study from a case-by-case perspective.

These guidelines should not be interpreted as ironclad rules for data analysis. During data analysis, you may find that keeping a log of what was done and why is helpful in directing the analysis of data in new, but organized directions. Review the log frequently. Writing summaries of the results of completed data analyses may also be a useful reference point. Review these summaries, discuss them with colleagues, and compare them with results of published research. Occasionally, reading about research that is unrelated but similar in design can be helpful in organizing and guiding the data analysis in new and meaningful directions.

We next demonstrate the use of quantitative data in statement synthesis. We will present a small segment of data from a nonexperimental study that one of us completed. (Data were gathered with support from grant number NU 00677, Division of Nursing, U.S. Public Health Service.) In one part of the study, attitudes and beliefs of new mothers were investigated. Because the literature suggested that maternal parity and infant sex might influence attitudes and beliefs, data were analyzed separately according to parity (primiparas and multiparas) and infant sex (male and female) subgroups. Although this division reduced the number of subjects within groups, it provided a sharper picture of attitudes or belief patterns among new mothers. Table 6–2 presents the correlations among three attitudes and beliefs measured at the beginning and at the end of the neonatal period. The correlations are presented for each of the four subgroups of new mothers. The correlations of mothers' attitudes toward themselves as mothers are quite high for all four subgroups ($r = 0.62$ to 0.77). Thus, you might claim that mothers' attitudes toward themselves as mothers do not undergo major changes during the neonatal period. That is, overall attitude toward oneself as mother was a relatively stable phenomenon across time regardless of parity or sex of infant.

TABLE 6–2   CORRELATION BETWEEN NEW MOTHERS' ATTITUDES OR BELIEFS AT THE BEGINNING AND END OF THE NEONATAL PERIOD

Maternal Parity/ Infant Sex	Beliefs About Baby	Attitude Toward Baby	Attitude/Belief Attitude Toward Self as Mother
Primiparous/Female	0.35[a] (28)	0.44[b] (31)	0.62[c] (31)
Primiparous/Male	0.41[b] (42)	0.44[b] (43)	0.66[c] (43)
Multiparous/Female	−0.06 (51)	0.69[c] (51)	0.67[c] (51)
Multiparous/Male	−0.12 (35)	0.23 (38)	0.77[c] (38)

Note: Numbers of subjects are in parentheses. These may vary within groups because of some missing data.
[a] = $p < .05$.
[b] = $p < .01$.
[c] = $p < .001$.

For beliefs about one's infant, however, this was not true. Beliefs about one's baby were significantly correlated across the neonatal period for primiparous mothers ($r = 0.35$ to 0.41), but not for multiparas ($r = -0.06$ to -0.12). Thus, beliefs about one's baby are somewhat stable for first-time mothers; for mothers having other than a first baby, beliefs at the end of the neonatal period are unrelated to initial beliefs.

This last finding was indeed surprising. You might have expected that inexperienced mothers would have unrealistic beliefs about infants so that they would be the group most likely to change their beliefs over the course of the neonatal period. What we speculate happened is this. First-time mothers, because of their inexperience with infants, "stereotype" them. Thus, when the infant's early behavior is different from expectations, these behaviors are ignored and the stereotype is maintained. Mothers who have already had at least one child have learned over time that babies are very individual as they compared their earlier babies' growth and behavior with other babies. Thus, "repeat" mothers did not expect babies to conform to a stereotype. As a result, repeat mothers change their initial beliefs about their later babies more readily than first-time mothers as they come to know their individual behaviors. Explanations other than this one, of course, may also be given for the surprising results reported here.

Now look at the column in Table 6–2 labeled "Attitude Toward Baby." Make a statement about how consistent across time mothers' attitudes toward their babies were for the four groups. Try to construct a reason that would explain the statement you made. In constructing your statement, you should have noted that mothers' attitudes toward their babies were significantly related across the neonatal period for all four groups of mothers ($r = 0.44$ to 0.69) except for multiparous mothers of male infants ($r = 0.23$). Several hypotheses explaining this finding may be offered. We hypothesize that mothers of firstborns stereotype their babies so that their attitudes remain somewhat consistent over time regardless of their infant's sex. Let us assume, however, that male infants as a group are more unpredictable or variable than females in the first weeks of life. If we further assume that multiparous mothers are more aware of individuality of infants, we might then expect that multiparous mothers of male infants might change their attitudes more than other mothers in response to the variability of their babies. Your reasons may be as plausible as the ones offered here. Given the limited information we have provided here, there is no single best explanation. Examining the available data would help to evaluate the plausibility of the explanation we have given here. For example, the data might be examined to determine if male infants were indeed more variable than females in the neonatal period.

It is important to remember that although we have given a number of guidelines for the analysis and interpretation of quantitative nonexperimental data, we have not stated exact procedures for the application of this method. We have avoided stating procedures because we did not want to mislead readers into believing that statement synthesis is a mechanical process of inspecting data and then simply formulating statements from the data. A key strategic aspect of statistically based statement synthesis is in the organization of the data analysis. We have tried to emphasize this aspect, being assured that research methods texts amply cover procedural aspects of quantitative nonexperimental research (Pedhazur & Schmelkin, 1991; Polit & Beck, 2003). We believe the information on strategic aspects of quantitative methods in a discovery context presented here is not addressed in conventional research texts.

Embedded in our presentation of quantitative methods has been a threefold process: (1) approach data analysis in inventive yet organized ways, (2) carefully describe results via systematic formulation of statements, and (3) where possible, link statements derived from data with existing theories or hypothesized explanations. Although the third phase moves beyond statement synthesis itself, it is meaningful to include it here to set the stage for other theoretical activities such as theory synthesis and theory testing.

Quantitative methods require the continuing and thoughtful attention of the theorist in the data analytic and interpretive processes, lest the theorist become lost in an array of numbers. Nonetheless, quantitative methods in general offer theorists the advantage of access to explicit numerical data about a phenomenon. Numbers may lack the flavor of reality, but they can aid relationship identification in ways the naked eye may miss. Statements of relationships are in the end an abstraction about reality, not reality itself. Quantitative methods can facilitate the abstraction process in that their application to reality forces a theorist to think about reality in conceptual and quantitative dimensions.

Literary Methods

Literary methods of statement synthesis start out with statements derived from extant research. In contrast to statement analysis, literary methods of statement synthesis utilize only those statements in scientific literature that are derived or supported by empirical evidence. Relationships that are conjectural on a theorist's part or that are not founded on research usually are not included. This criterion for statement inclusion does not necessarily mean that conjectures or unsupported statements are useless in theory construction. Rather, the criterion reflects the orientation of synthesis strategies: to begin theoretical work from empirical evidence. Conjectural or unsupported statements fail to meet this criterion. Conjectural statements may be useful, however, in other types of strategies, such as statement analysis or statement derivation.

To illustrate the process of statement synthesis, we examine a classic study conducted by Henthorn (1979). The following statement was empirically supported in Henthorn's study of disengagement and reinforcement in the elderly:

> the greater the degree of disengagement [reported by the elderly], the lower the level of reinforcement [of role behaviors by others] and the anticipated reinforcement [of role behaviors by others]. (p. 5)

Often statements such as this need to be rewritten to clarify their meaning. In this example, the statement in fact describes two sets of relationships, which may be restated as follows:

the greater the degree of disengagement reported by the elderly, the lower the level of reinforcement of role behaviors by others.

and

the greater the degree of disengagement reported by the elderly, the lower the anticipated reinforcement of role behaviors by others.

There are several equivalent forms in which relational statements such as those above may be written:

The greater the X, the greater the Y.

As X increases (or decreases), Y increases (or decreases).

X and Y covary.

X is positively (or negatively) related to Y.

The form in which these statements are written is ambiguous. Left open are several questions:

1. Is the relationship between X and Y reversible; that is, if an increase in X is related to an increase in Y, is an increase in Y also related to an increase in X?
2. Is the relationship between the two variables X and Y causal or noncausal (simply associative)?

These questions can be answered only if the design of the research from which the statement was derived was aimed at disentangling these issues. Otherwise, the theorist must simply recognize the ambiguity and await further research that can clarify the answers to the reversibility and causality questions.

Experimental approaches and in some cases longitudinal data can help clarify questions left ambiguous by correlational or nonexperimental designs. Where answers to questions about causality and reversibility can be answered, the form in which statements may be written is more precise. For example,

Only if there is an increase in X, will there be an increase in Y, but the reverse is not true (nonreversible or unidirectional causality),

or

Only if there is an increase in X, will there be an increase in Y, and vice versa (reversibility or bidirectional causality).

Two techniques are involved in literary statement synthesis: (1) making the meanings of the concepts included in a statement more general, or (2) expanding the boundaries (scope of phenomena covered) to include a wider variety of situations. The first may be done by merging less general concepts into a more abstract, general concept. The latter is done by reformulating the boundaries of a statement to increase the populations and situations to which it applies; for example, extending statements about small group-interaction patterns to all groups regardless of size. We will apply both of these techniques of literary synthesis. Our first revised statement taken from Henthorn will be the starting point:

> *The greater the degree of disengagement reported by the elderly, the lower the level of reinforcement of role behaviors by others.*

Now let us take a statement from Osofsky and Danzger's (1974) important research on early mother–infant interaction. They noted that

> *the attentive mother tends to have a responsive baby and vice versa. (p. 124)*

To synthesize the statements from Henthorn's (1979) and Osofsky and Danzger's (1974) studies, we first need to develop a broader concept from the concepts "degree of disengagement" and "attentive mother." Common to these two concepts is a more general concept: "amount of socially interactive behaviors an individual displays." For the concepts "level of reinforcement of role behaviors by others" and "responsive baby," a commonality exists in the higher order concept "social reinforcement that accompanies socially interactive behaviors." We further broaden the situational scope of our statement by shifting the boundaries from the elderly or mothers and infants to an individual in social interaction with others. Thus, a synthesized statement drawn from Henthorn's and Osofsky and Danzger's studies may be made.

> *The amount of socially interactive behaviors an individual displays is directly related to the amount of social reinforcement received from others.*

Finally, because we were unclear about the reversibility of Henthorn's statement, we chose a conservative interpretation of it and wrote the synthesized statement as nonreversible.

In the example of social interaction and reinforcement we have tried to show how a general statement may be synthesized from two statements that initially appear dissimilar. This was done to help the reader grasp the basic, and sometimes surprising, ways in which research outcomes can be pulled together into synthesized statements. Formulating a statement that generalizes to new and broader boundaries, of course, requires that additional data be sought to substantiate the new generalization. Nonetheless, an important move in theory construction may have been made as further evidence is being awaited.

Now let's turn to actual examples of statement synthesis in nursing. This strategy has been shown to be useful in the process of building middle-range prescriptive theories in nursing. For example, statement synthesis has been cited as a component of prescriptive theory building related to the following clinical concerns: balance between analgesia and side effects in adults (Good & Moore, 1996); peaceful end of life (Ruland & Moore, 1998); and acute pain management in infants and children (Huth & Moore, 1998). In each of these three theory-building efforts, existing bodies of clinical knowledge gathered together in the form of either clinical guidelines or standards of practice were transformed into middle-range theories using the strategies of statement synthesis and then theory synthesis. An example of using statement synthesis to develop relational statements for such theories is well illustrated by Ruland and Moore's (1998) work in developing a statement related to patient comfort in end-of-life care.

First, Ruland and Moore (1998) examined 16 outcome criteria for standards of practice related to peaceful end of life developed by nursing experts in Norway. These 16 outcome criteria were then restated as five higher order concepts (called "outcome indicators"), one of which was "the experience of comfort" (p. 172). Thirteen specific process criteria within the standards related to the experience of comfort were identified and restated in terms of three higher order nursing interventions (called "prescriptors"). For example, one of three prescriptors was "preventing, monitoring, and relieving physical discomfort" (p. 173). The resulting synthesized statement including all three prescriptors was expressed as follows:

> *Preventing, monitoring, and relieving physical discomfort, facilitating rest, relaxation, and contentment, and preventing complications contribute to the patient's experience of comfort. (p. 174)*

Ruland and Moore synthesized a total of six relational statements that then served as the statemental components in their subsequent theory synthesis.

Literary methods of statement synthesis may be given a still further level of precision. Where a series of statements has been synthesized from research literature on a phenomenon, statements may be ranked or classified according to the level of empirical support available to substantiate them, such as strong consistent support; moderate support; and low inconsistent support. Statements that have supporting evidence collected in multiple studies using diverse populations would be ranked higher than those with a more limited base of evidence. Particularly where research findings are used as a basis for public policy formation or for application to practice, clear determination of the extent of support for synthesized statements is important.

Literary statement synthesis, although time consuming, involves minimal cost and resources compared to other statement synthesis methods. Access to adequate library facilities is crucial to this method. Literary approaches to statement synthesis are especially useful in that statements generated are not limited to the findings of any one study. Access to findings of multiple studies on a topic of interest offers a richer database than any single study. Literary approaches will be only partly satisfactory, however, where the published research on a topic is limited in amount and quality.

ADVANTAGES AND LIMITATIONS

Because methods of statement synthesis are so varied, we will speak to advantages and limitations in only the most general terms here. An evaluation of the advantages and limitations of statement synthesis methods as a group hinges on philosophical assumptions that are discussed below.

Statement synthesis as a method assumes that confrontation with reality is a useful and productive means of constructing theory. It assumes that without the aid of a clear guiding theory, a theorist can detect the dimensions of a phenomenon that are the most scientifically useful. In describing such atheoretical approaches to theory construction as "research-then-theory," Reynolds (1971) noted that they assume there are real patterns that exist in nature. These patterns are then discovered by researchers using empirical methods. In this viewpoint, "research" is akin to "search." Reynolds further notes that the assumptions made about how scientific knowledge relates to the real world are philosophical and thus not amenable to resolution by scientific methods. We must leave our readers to decide for themselves, using philosophical methods, if they find the assumptions of synthetic methods tenable. This issue goes beyond the scope of this book. We hope that readers will find these philosophical issues as intriguing as the more procedural ones treated in this book.

UTILIZING THE RESULTS OF STATEMENT SYNTHESIS

The aim of statement synthesis is to formulate statements about nursing phenomena from observations (both qualitatively and quantitatively recorded) and from published evidence. Utilizing the results of this strategy leads directly into the larger knowledge-generating process. Thus, this strategy forms the substance of evidence-based practice. It also is employed in reviewing research literature as a preamble to a study, reaching study conclusions, and transmitting those conclusions through the educational process. If the practicing nurse, researcher, and teacher are committed to carefully grounding their work on scientific observation, then statement synthesis is not a product used, but rather a process at the heart of what each does. Statement synthesis may also be a bridge to theory synthesis (see Chapter 9).

Statements carefully formulated from research and observation can be helpful, particularly in undergraduate nursing education. Although concept teaching may provide the foci of nursing content, only when concepts are linked within statements do explanations and predictions become possible. The latter form the base for making logical inferences in relating content to practice. Thus, synthesized statements may be used to enrich the content of nursing instruction.

SUMMARY

Statement synthesis is an empirically based strategy for constructing statements that specify the manner in which two or more concepts are interrelated. The strategy encompasses a number of diverse approaches to developing statements. Specific methods range from direct observation and analysis (qualitative or quantitative) of data to use of accumulated research-based literature to construct higher order generalizations.

Qualitative methods rely on theorists to be perceptive of processes that underlie the events they confront in the data gathering and analysis. Quantitative approaches begin with identifying numerical ways of observing reality. These are then analyzed with the aid of statistical methods to sharpen the patterns inherent in data. Literary methods aim at pulling together general statements of relationships from available research. Despite the diversity of these methods, they share in common a dependence on evidence for formulating scientific statements and a common philosophical assumption about how scientific knowledge reflects reality.

PRACTICE EXERCISES

In Table 6–3 we present a continuation of the study of new mothers' beliefs and attitudes reported earlier in this chapter. The information addresses the relationship of attitudes toward the baby and attitudes toward oneself as mother as each of these relate to beliefs about the baby. The correlations between these measures were based on data collected at the end of the neonatal period. As before, the correlations are reported separately by parity and sex groups.

Look carefully at the information in Table 6–3. Formulate one or more statements about how sex and parity groups are similar or different in terms of relationships reported. Formulate an explanation for the results as you stated them.

After inspecting the data you should have noted that for all mothers, except multiparous mothers of males, beliefs about one's baby and attitude toward one's baby were significantly correlated. However, beliefs about one's baby and attitude

TABLE 6–3   CORRELATION BETWEEN NEW MOTHERS' ATTITUDES AND BELIEFS AT THE END OF THE NEONATAL PERIOD

	Correlation Among Attitudes and Beliefs[a]	
Maternal Parity/ Infant Sex	**Beliefs About Baby and Attitude Toward Baby**	**Beliefs About Baby and Attitude Toward Self as Mother**
Primiparous/Female	-0.59^{b} (28)	-0.67^{b} (28)
Primiparous/Male	-0.50^{b} (43)	-0.26 (43)
Multiparous/Female	-0.39^{c} (49)	0.14 (49)
Multiparous/Male	-0.28 (34)	-0.13 (34)

Note: Number of subjects are in parentheses.
[a]The negative sign (-0.00) on the correlations is an artifact of the opposite direction in which the attitude and belief scales are scored; for this exercise the negative sign on the correlations may be ignored and the correlations treated essentially as positive relations among variables.
[b] $= p < .001$.
[c] $= p < .01$.

toward oneself as mother were uncorrelated within all groups except primiparous mothers of girls.

Because we have earlier offered explanations for the unique features of the relationship of a multiparous mother and her male infant, we will not repeat those here. That line of reasoning would help to explain the pattern of correlations between beliefs about the baby and attitude toward baby.

Regarding the correlation patterns of parity and sex groups for beliefs about baby and attitude toward self as mother, we hypothesize the following. Mothers construct worldviews of themselves and how they relate to their infants. The mothers' attitude toward themselves may either be integrated with their beliefs about their babies or distinct from them. Where mothers are confident in themselves, their views of themselves will be distinct or separate from how they see their infants. Also, where mothers hold beliefs about their babies that are many times proven wrong, they will also tend to separate their beliefs about their babies from their attitude toward themselves. Multiparous mothers are likely to view their babies separately from themselves because of their confidence in themselves as successful mothers in the past. For different reasons, such as unpredictable behavior of the male infant, primiparous mothers of males will also separate their beliefs about their infants from their attitude toward themselves as mothers. Only first-time mothers of females do not differentiate their attitude toward themselves from their beliefs about their infants.

As before, your explanation may be as plausible as the one offered here. What is most important, however, is that you now should be able to look at data, describe it, and hypothesize about reasons behind it.

SELF-ASSESSMENT TEST OF INTRODUCTORY STATISTICS

For readers who wish to assess or refresh their knowledge of introductory statistics to maximally benefit from this chapter, the following self-assessment test is provided. Answers are given at the end of the chapter following the References and Additional Readings sections.

1. Overall, the best predictor of any individual's score on a test is the
   A. variance.
   B. standard deviation.
   C. correlation.
   D. mean.

2. Changing an individual's raw scores on several tests into percentages has what effect?
   A. splits an individual score into quartiles
   B. locks an individual's scores into a common unit
   C. establishes the group mean
   D. results in the calculation of the group variance

3. The x^2 statistic is designed to analyze data that are
    A. categorical (noncontinuous).
    B. ordinal (rank-ordered).
    C. interval (equal interval).
    D. ratio (true zero point).

4. A correlation coefficient reflects the
    A. average deviation from the mean.
    B. difference between two means.
    C. relationship between two variables.
    D. most frequently occurring score in a score distribution.

5. A t test and analysis of variance (ANOVA) are similar in that both
    A. apply to categorical data.
    B. test the differences between means.
    C. test the relationship between variables.
    D. may be used to compute the variance.

6. Nurse A collected information on which patients kept or broke their clinic appointments during one month. Further, Nurse A classified all these patients as "teenagers" or "nonteenagers" to determine if teenagers had special problems in keeping appointments. To analyze Nurse A's data, the most appropriate statistic is which of the following?
    A. measure of central tendency
    B. x^2
    C. correlated t test
    D. analysis of variance

7. In analyzing some other data about clinic patients, Nurse A calculated a correlation coefficient of $+2.19$. The size of the correlation indicates
    A. a strong relationship.
    B. a large difference.
    C. a significant finding.
    D. an error in calculation.

8. The director of the clinic told Nurse A that evidence was needed to show the effectiveness of the patient education done in the clinic. Nurse A decided to compare hypertensive patients' systolic blood pressures before and after the patient education program 1 year ago. To do this, Nurse A should use which test statistic?
    A. a measure of deviation from the mean
    B. x^2
    C. correlation
    D. t test

Answers of Self-Assessment Test of Introductory Statistics

1. D; 2. B; 3. A; 4. C; 5. B; 6. B; 7. D; 8. D

REFERENCES

Aiken LR. *Rating Scales and Checklists: Evaluating Behavior, Personality, and Attitudes.* New York, NY: Wiley; 1996.

Anastasi A. *Psychological Testing.* 7th ed. Upper Saddle River, NJ: Prentice Hall; 1997.

Benoliel JQ. Grounded theory and nursing knowledge. *Qual Health Res.* 1996;6:406-428.

Cronbach LJ. *Essentials of Psychological Testing.* 5th ed. Reading, Mass: Addison-Wesley; 1997.

Cronbach LJ, Meehl PE. Construct validity in psychological tests. In: Jackson DN, Messick S, eds. *Problems in Human Assessment.* New York, NY: McGraw-Hill; 1967.

Denzin NK, Lincoln YS. *Handbook of Qualitative Research.* 2nd ed. Thousand Oaks, Calif: Sage Publications; 2000.

Eaves YD. A synthesis technique for grounded theory data analysis. *J Adv Nurs.* 2001; 35:654-663.

Glaser BG. *Theoretical Sensitivity.* Mill Valley, Calif: Sociology Press; 1978.

Glaser BG, Strauss AL. *The Discovery of Grounded Theory: Strategies for Qualitative Research.* Chicago, Ill: Aldine; 1967.

Good M, Moore SM. Clinical practice guidelines as a new source of middle-range theory: focus on acute pain. *Nurs Outlook.* 1996;44:74-79.

Henthorn BS. Disengagement and reinforcement in the elderly. *Res Nurs Health.* 1979;2:1-8.

Huth MM, Moore SM. Prescriptive theory of acute pain management in infants and children. *J Soc Pediatr Nurses.* 1998;3:23-32.

Kiernan M, King AC, Kraemer HC, Stefanick ML, Killen JD. Characteristics of successful and unsuccessful dieters: an application of signal detection methodology. *Ann Behav Med.* 1998;20:1-6.

Knafl KA, Grace HK, eds. *Families Across the Life Cycle.* Boston, Mass: Little, Brown; 1978.

Nunnally JC, Bernstein IH. *Psychometric Theory.* 3rd ed. Burr Ridge, Ill: McGraw-Hill; 1994.

Osofsky JD, Danzger B. Relationships between neonatal characteristics and mother-infant interaction. *Devel Psychol.* 1974;10:124-130.

Pedhazur EJ, Schmelkin LP. *Measurement, Design, and Analysis: An Integrated Approach.* Hillsdale, NJ: Erlbaum; 1991.

Polit DF, *Data Analysis & Statistics for Nursing Research.* Stamford, Conn: Appleton & Lange; 1996.

Polit DF, Beck CT. *Nursing Research: Principles and Methods.* 7th ed. Philadelphia, Penn: Lippincott; 2003.

Quint JC. The case for theories generated from empirical data. *Nurs Res.* 1967a;16:109-114.

Quint JC. *The Nurse and the Dying Patient.* New York, NY: Macmillan; 1967b.

Reynolds PD. *A Primer in Theory Construction.* Indianapolis, Ind: Bobbs-Merrill; 1971.

Ruland CM, Moore SM. Theory construction based on standards of care: a proposed theory of the peaceful end of life. *Nurs Outlook.* 1998; 46:169-175.

Schatzman L, Strauss AL. *Field Research: Strategies for a Natural Sociology.* Englewood Cliffs, NJ: Prentice Hall; 1973.

Schreiber RS, Stern PN. *Using Grounded Theory in Nursing.* New York, NY: Springer; 2001.

Stern PN. Grounded theory methodology: its uses and processes. *Image.* 1980;12:20-23.

Strauss A, Corbin JM. *Basics of Qualitative Research: Techniques and Procedures for Developing Grounded Theory.* Thousand Oaks, Calif: Sage Publications; 1998.

Tabachnick BG, Fidell LS. *Using Multivariate Statistics.* 4th ed. Boston, Mass: Allyn & Bacon; 2001.
Waltz CF, Strickland OL, Lenz ER. *Measurement in Nursing Research.* 2nd ed. Philadelphia, Penn: Davis; 1991.

ADDITIONAL READINGS
Readings in Statistics

Readers who want more information on statistics may find some of the texts below of interest.

Hays WL. *Statistics.* 5th ed. Fort Worth, Tex: Harcourt, Brace, Jovanovich College; 1993.
Heiman GW. *Understanding Research Methods and Statistics.* 2nd ed. Boston, Mass: Houghton Mifflin; 2001.
Newton RR, Rudestam KE. *Your Statistical Consultant: Answers to Your Data Analysis Questions.* Thousand Oaks, Calif: Sage Publications; 1999.
Polit DF. *Data Analysis & Statistics for Nursing Research.* Stamford, Conn: Appleton & Lange; 1996.
Tabachnick BG, Fidell LS. *Using Multivariate Statistics.* 4th ed. Boston, Mass: Allyn & Bacon; 2001.
Vernoy M, Kyle D. *Behavioral Statistics in Action.* Boston, Mass: McGraw-Hill; 2002.
Williams F. *Reasoning with Statistics.* 5th ed. San Diego, Calif: Harcourt; 2000.

Readings in Statement Construction

Readers who want more information on statement construction may find some of the classic texts below of interest.

Dubin R. *Theory Building.* New York, NY: Free Press; 1978.
Hage J. *Techniques and Problems of Theory Construction in Sociology.* New York, NY: Wiley; 1972.
Mullins NC. *The Art of Theory: Construction and Use.* New York, NY: Harper & Row; 1971.
Olson S. *Ideas and Data: The Process and Practice of Social Research.* Homewood, Ill: Dorsey; 1976.
Pillemer DB, Light RJ. Synthesizing outcomes: how to use research evidence from many studies. *Harvard Educ Rev.* 1980;50:176-195.
Reynolds PD. *A Primer in Theory Construction.* Indianapolis, Ind: Bobbs-Merrill; 1971.
Zetterberg HL. *On Theory and Verification in Sociology.* Totowa, NJ: Bedminister Press; 1965.

7

Statement Derivation

Preliminary Note: *Like concept derivation, statement derivation is one of the less frequently used strategies, based on formal citations in articles. Nevertheless, it is foundational in the larger process of theory derivation, a more frequently used strategy. As a result, a firm grasp of this strategy is useful to readers who wish to pursue theory derivation activities, or who wish simply to understand the process of statement formulation with greater clarity.*

DEFINITION AND DESCRIPTION

Statement derivation is a strategy for developing a set of statements about a phenomenon by using an analogy. Statement derivation draws on the earlier work of Maccia and Maccia (1963) on educational theorizing through models. A set of statements (S_1) from one field of interest (F_1) is used to derive the content or structure of a second set of statements (S_2) for a second field (F_2). Thus, a second series of statements is created that shares some common structural or content features with an existing set of statements. Despite similar structure or terminology, the two sets of statements are distinct because each refers to a separate field of interest (see Figure 7–1).

Identifying an analogy or likeness between phenomena in two different fields is the basis of statement derivation. The likeness or analogy between statements in two fields may be either substantive or formal. In a substantive analogy the likeness rests in the content or concepts in two fields. In a formal analogy it is the logical structure linking together concepts in one field that is analogous to or like a second field. On the surface, the two fields of interest do not necessarily have to appear similar. What is required is that there be analogous dimensions between phenomena in the two fields. For example, let us assume the following statement holds true in physical science: For any two objects in motion close to each other, there are forces that attract the objects to each other as well as forces that repel them. By analogy, we might theorize that for any two persons who are in close physical contact with each other, there are forces that attract the persons to each

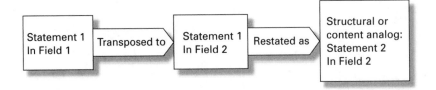

FIGURE 7–1 Process of statement derivation.

other as well as forces that repel them. Despite gross differences in the phenomena in the two fields, these two statements bear a structural and content similarity to each other.

The processes for deriving the content and structure of statements are crucial to understanding statement derivation. Deriving the *content* and *structure* of a new statement from an existing source or parent statement involves two logically separate derivations. Whereas a theorist might simultaneously carry out the content and structural aspects of statement derivation, we will separate them to present each aspect more clearly.

Derivation of the content of a new statement is akin to concept derivation (see Chapter 4). What a theorist does is specify the terms or concepts to be included in a new statement and their accompanying definitions within the new field. Derivation of the structure of the new statements entails specifying the type of linkage between the newly derived concepts or terms. The linkage may be a unidirectional causal relationship, a simple positive relationship, a negative association, or a more complex algebraic relationship. (See Chapter 8 for an analysis of the types of linkages between the concepts in statements.)

Let's look at the following sample statement that will be used to derive a statement about family interaction.

> When the volume of a gas is held constant, the temperature and pressure are positively related.

Content derivation focuses on specifying family terminology to parallel the key chemical concepts or terms in this statement: *gas, volume, temperature,* and *pressure.* For example, the terms *family, amount of interaction, amount of hostile comments,* and *amount of angry responses* might be defined as respective analogs of the chemical terminology.

In looking at the structural derivation of a new statement, content terms that refer to the properties of the phenomenon, for example, *pressure,* may be eliminated and replaced by simple placeholding symbols such as *A, B,* and *C*. Thus, our beginning statement may be rewritten as follows:

When the A of a B is held constant, the C and D are positively related.

This noncontent statement presents only the skeleton or structure of relationships among our unspecified concepts or terms *A, B, C,* and *D*. As written, the statement makes logical sense but does not have any meaning in terms of real phenomena. Until *A–D* are given substance by terms linking them to reality, the statement is not empirically interpretable. To specify meanings for *A–D*, let us substitute the terms developed earlier for family interaction.

When the amount of interaction of a family is held constant, the amount of hostile comments and the amount of angry responses are positively related.

Not all cases of statement derivation need entail both content and structural derivation aspects. If a theorist has already delineated relevant concepts describing a phenomenon and lacks only a clear mode of interrelating them, only the structural aspect of statement derivation may be needed.

Parallels in the structure or content of statements across fields are based on the analogy that a theorist identifies as implicit between two fields of interest. As a result, a large measure of the success of statement derivation hinges on the theorist's insightful selection of an existing field that contains rich parallels with the theorist's field of interest. There is no set rule for selecting timely and fruitful source or parent fields from which to begin statement derivation. A theorist's "sense" or awareness of phenomena in the field of interest is certainly an important ingredient. Reading in fields that are related as well as unrelated to the theorist's interests also can establish a range of alternate fields from which to begin statement derivation. The true heuristic value of a parent field can be determined only as a theorist actually attempts to derive statements from a parent field.

PURPOSE AND USES

The purpose of statement derivation is to formulate one or more statements about a phenomenon that is currently not well understood. Statement derivation is especially suited to situations in which (1) no available database or body of literature exists, or (2) current thinking is becoming outmoded and new perspectives are needed. Statement derivation is especially relevant when a theorist wishes to clarify how several dimensions of a phenomenon are related, or wants a derived set of statements about a phenomenon in order to then build an integrated theoretical model of it. For example, suppose a theorist wished to clarify how telephone support from a clinical nurse specialist affects men's coping after surgery for prostate cancer. A literature search of CINAHL showed the theorist that there were only a few articles about the role of the clinical nurse specialist (CNS) and care of patients with prostate cancer (Higgins, 2000). Furthermore, a search of Medline showed that most studies of telephone support were focused mainly on men undergoing radiation therapy for prostate or bladder cancer (e.g., Faithfull, Corner, Meyer, Huddart, & Dearnaley,

2001; Rose, Shrader-Bogen, Korlath, Priem, & Larson, 1996). The nurse theorist concluded that statement development in this important area of cancer care was needed. Statement derivation appeared to be the most reasonable and rapid means of developing one or more statements about telephone support from a CNS and resultant postsurgical coping of men with prostate cancer. We will continue with the example of CNS telephone support in the next section.

PROCEDURES FOR STATEMENT DERIVATION

Statement derivation may be broken down into several steps. In actual practice, a theorist may move through several steps almost simultaneously or occasionally repeat steps to improve the final results. The steps are, thus, guideposts rather than rigid lock-step maneuvers in statement building. Bearing this in mind, we list the steps in statement derivation below.

1. Become thoroughly familiar with any existing literature on a topic of interest. This should involve not only reading but also critically evaluating the level of usefulness of statements about the topic of interest. This step should determine the need to use the statement derivation strategy. If a need for a new perspective is evident, or a paucity of relevant literature is available, then statement derivation may be appropriate.
2. Search other fields for new ways of looking at the topic of interest. Read literature from several fields, some similar to and some dissimilar from the topic and field of interest. Be alert to those aspects of the literature that specifically express the major relational statements of each field.
3. Select the source or parent field to be used in the derivation process, and carefully identify the structural and content features of the parent statements to be used in derivations. Be sure to separately consider both the structural suitability and the content suitability of statements in the parent field. Because derivation is not a mechanical process, the theorist is free to modify statements in the parent field to increase their suitability to the derivation process. Thus, statements from the parent field may be restated to enhance their clarity and to more sharply display the structure of relationships between concepts.
4. Develop new statements about the topic of interest from the content and structure of statements in the parent field. This step, simply stated, consists of restating the parent statements in terms of the subject matter of the new field, that is, the theorist's topic of interest.
5. Redefine any new concepts or terms in the derived statements to fit the specific subject matter of the topic of interest. If statement derivation is used only to provide the structure for interrelating concepts that already exist in the field of interest, much of this step may already be done. Even so, it is prudent to reassess the suitability of definitions of terms when they are placed within the structure of new statements. Adaptations in meaning may be needed.

To illustrate these steps in operation, we will continue to explore the hypothetical case of the nurse theorist interested in CNS telephone support and its relationship to men's coping after surgery for prostate cancer. For this illustration, the theorist had already identified the two concepts of "CNS telephone support" and "postsurgical coping" as the concepts of interest. Thus, only a structural linkage between the two concepts needed to be specified in the statement derivation. In searching other fields for analogous ways of viewing the CNS–patient telephone interaction, the theorist located literature on the inverted U function. In psychological literature independent variables such as anxiety are related to outcomes such as performance in a curvilinear or inverted U form. Thus, high and low levels of anxiety are related to less effective performance whereas moderate levels of anxiety are associated with high levels of performance. The inverted U function has proven to be useful in other fields such as interactions between mothers and high-risk infants (Field, 1980). The nurse theorist therefore chose the inverted U function as the structure for a statement about CNS telephone support and patient coping. In applying the inverted U function to the concepts of interest, the following statement was derived.

> *CNS telephone support is related to patient postsurgical coping as an inverted U function: high and low levels of CNS telephone support are related to low patient coping whereas moderate levels of CNS telephone support are related to high levels of patient coping.*

The inverted U function between CNS telephone support and patient coping is depicted in Figure 7–2.

To complete the statement development process, the theorist then prepared definitions of CNS telephone support and postsurgical coping with prostate cancer. The theorist also operationally defined high, medium, and low levels of CNS telephone support based on the literature.

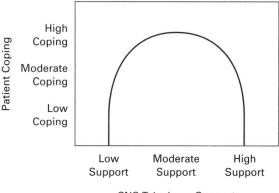

FIGURE 7–2   Hypothetical relationship of CNS telephone support to patient coping after prostate surgery for cancer.

The theorist in our illustration of CNS telephone support utilized only the structural aspect of statement derivation. Because the content concepts were already identified, only a structure for interrelating them was needed. This was provided by the inverted U function. When theorists are deriving *both* the content and structure of a new statement, the derivation process will more closely resemble the example of family-interaction patterns presented earlier in this chapter.

The derived statement about CNS telephone support predicts how support is related to patient coping. However, the empirical validity of this or any other derived statements cannot be known before testing. Testing the accuracy of derived statements is quite important to practice. Testing is needed to see if low, moderate, and high levels of CNS telephone support are indeed related to patient coping as an inverted U function. If confirmed by research, the statement is relevant to evidence-based approaches to practice. (*Note:* The example of CNS telephone support for postoperative patients with prostate cancer is presented for illustrative purposes and should not be construed as a definitive review on this topic.)

An initial way of assessing the potential plausibility of derived statements is to examine existing research literature for supporting evidence. Perhaps studies not directly aimed at testing the effects of CNS telephone support contain data that are relevant to the statement in question. Perhaps related research has been done in other areas of cancer care. These data, although not a direct test of the support–coping statement, add to its plausibility or nonplausibility. Finally, if highly regarded theories are found to predict the inverted U function between CNS telephone support and coping, a further measure of support is given to the statement. None of the methods outlined here is a substitute for definitive testing of a derived statement, but each aids in making a provisional estimate of the statement's plausibility.

Ultimately, however, derived statements must be tested to determine their credibility. Such testing is essential before derived statements can be applied to practice. A lengthy discussion of statement testing is outside the focus of this chapter. Readers may consult research methods texts for information about appropriate research designs for testing interventions and related clinical questions (Cook & Campbell, 1979; Kerlinger, 1986; Pedhazur & Schmelkin, 1991; Polit & Beck, 2003). Statement testing is also briefly covered in Chapter 12.

Finally, theorists should not begin evaluating the empirical support for a statement before they have come to closure on the derivation process. Prematurely evaluating the plausibility of a statement may close off the theorist's creative processes. Even in the early stages of derivation when a theorist is selecting parent statements, these should not be stringently judged, but simply examined and toyed with. Sometimes seemingly unlikely candidates may prove to be winners in the long run. We are reminded of Maccia and Maccia's (1963) use of the physiology of eye blinking as a framework for deriving statements about student learning. Although judging has its place in the context of justification, it should be held in abeyance in the context of discovery (see Chapter 1).

ADVANTAGES AND LIMITATIONS

As a strategy, statement derivation offers two advantages. The strategy is an economical and expeditious way of developing statements about a phenomenon. Unlike statement synthesis, the strategy does not require data as a starting point. Armed with only an idea of the phenomenon of interest, reference materials from other fields, and a measure of creative ability, a theorist can accomplish statement derivation. The strategy is not limited to any discipline or phenomenon. It may be used with whatever subject matter a theorist chooses.

Statement derivation also has a serious limitation. Derivation of new statements from credible statements in another field of scholarship does not lend support directly to the newly derived statements. Even though derivation may facilitate development of interesting new scientific statements, independent empirical support of derived statements is still required.

UTILIZING THE RESULTS OF STATEMENT DERIVATION

Statements constructed through the derivation process are essentially untested, thus, their most suitable application is in directing research efforts to test them. We see two noteworthy areas of research particularly suited for testing derived statements: (1) correlational studies to assess the relationship of an antecedent to a clinical phenomenon and (2) experimental studies to test the usefulness of a nursing intervention to ameliorate a clinical problem. Research methods texts that may be helpful to readers in statement testing are cited earlier in this chapter. To estimate the provisional empirical support for a derived statement, existing research findings often offer clues. For example, correlational data from other studies can sometimes provide information about whether proposed antecedents of clinical phenomena really occur. By examining existing data tables in published research, such provisional evidence can often be located. If found, it supports the need for a research study to directly test the derived statements.

Statement derivation also may serve as a useful instructional strategy. As a classroom exercise for students, it can be used as the means of generating research hypotheses when students are beginning to learn the research process. Often students get caught up in the details of each specific research topic. Statement derivation offers a means of involving students in joint classroom exercises that free them to think more broadly about phenomena that concern nursing.

SUMMARY

Statement derivation employs an analogy as a basis for constructing new statements about a phenomenon. The theorist selects a parent field as the base for statement development. Analogs to the field to be described are identified. These may occur in the content or structure of derived statements. There are no exact rules for locating fruitful parent fields to use in derivation.

Statement derivation involves becoming familiar with and critiquing literature on the topic of interest, searching for a parent field, identifying content and structural features in parent statements, developing analogous content and structure for derived statements, and redefining new concepts within the new field of interest. Derived statements require testing independent of the discovery context to establish their empirical validity. As a strategy, statement derivation is economical and expeditious.

PRACTICE EXERCISES

To practice statement derivation, we have selected source or parent statements from a variety of fields. Included among these are some classic statements from the fields of learning and biology. Before trying to do any derivations with them, identify the phenomenon you would like to derive new statements about. Select one or more of the statements below as a parent statement. Identify the content and structural aspects of the parent statement. Develop the content and structural analogs of the derived statement. Redefine, if needed, any new concepts in the derived statements.

Statements from Several Disciplines

1. "Adaptation to life with a chronic illness is facilitated by a network of interpersonal relationships" (Chrisler & O'Hea, 2000, p. 330).
2. "The more frequently we have made a given response to a given stimulus, the more likely we are to make that response to that stimulus again" (Hill, 1985, pp. 30–31).
3. "Organisms are surviving because they are adapted, and they are adapted because they are surviving" (Burnett & Eisner, 1964, p. v).
4. "Neutral events that accompany or precede established negative reinforcements become negatively reinforcing" (Skinner, 1953, p. 173).
5. "Change occurs in little explosions in which matter is created and destroyed" (Wheeler, 2001, p. 41).
6. "By the preservation of constancy of the internal environment, warm-blooded animals are freed from the influence of vicissitudes in the external environment" (Cannon, 1963, p. 178).
7. "Blinking functions to protect the eye from contact and to rest the retina and the ocular muscles" (Maccia & Maccia, 1963, p. 34).
8. "The constant bombing of the pancreas by . . . huge hits of sugars and fats can eventually wear out the organ's insulin-producing 'islets'. . . " (Critser, 2001, p. 146).

Here are two examples. First, beginning with statement 7, Maccia and Maccia (1963) derived the following statement about educational processes:

Distraction functions to protect from *mental stress* and to rest from *mental effort*. (p. 34)

Words in *italics* constitute content derivations, whereas words not italicized represent derived structural forms within which content concepts are located.

For our second example, we selected statement 6 for the derivation exercise that follows. Our wish was to describe the individual's strengths in a social context. We defined the structure of statement 6 as follows:

> By the preservation of constancy of A, Bs are freed from the influence of C.

We defined the content terms *A–C* as follows: *A* is self-esteem, *Bs* are human beings, and *C* is social stressors. By inserting our content terms within the structural form, the following new statement was derived:

> By the preservation of constancy of self-esteem, human beings are freed from the influence of social stressors.

If you chose to use statement 6 in your derivations, your content concepts may be quite different from the ones we used.

Compare your derived statements with these examples. Although there are no right or wrong derivations, you should be able to identify the content and structural aspects of your derivations and see if they parallel the examples given here. If your derived statements look at all plausible, try to find literature that supports the statements. If you wish, map out a plan for empirically testing your statements.

REFERENCES

Burnett AL, Eisner T. *Animal Adaptation*. New York, NY: Holt, Rinehart & Winston; 1964.

Cannon WB. *The Wisdom of the Body*. New York, NY: Norton; 1963.

Cook TD, Campbell DT. *Quasi-Experimentation: Design and Analysis Issues for Field Settings*. Boston, Mass: Houghton Mifflin; 1979.

Chrisler JC, O'Hea EL. Gender, culture, and autoimmune disorders. In: Eisler RM, Hersen M, eds. *Handbook of Gender, Culture, and Health*. Mahwah, NJ: Erlbaum; 2000:321-342.

Critser G. Let them eat fat. In: Ferris T, ed. *The Best American Science Writing 2001*. New York, NY: HarperCollins; 2001:143-153.

Faithfull S, Corner J, Meyer L, Huddart R, Dearnaley D. Evaluation of nurse-led follow up for patients undergoing pelvic radiotherapy. *Br J Cancer*. 2001;85:1853-1864.

Field TM. Interactions of high-risk infants: quantitative and qualitative differences. In: Sawin DB, Hawkins RC, Walker LO, Penticuff JH, eds. *Exceptional Infant*. Vol. 4. *Psychosocial Risks in Infant–Environment Transactions*. New York, NY: Brunner/Mazel; 1980:120-143.

Higgins D. The role of the prostate cancer nurse specialist. *Prof Nurse*. 2000;15:539-542.

Hill WF. *Learning: A Survey of Psychological Interpretations*. 4th ed. New York, NY: Harper & Row; 1985.

Kerlinger FN. *Foundations of Behavioral Research*. 3rd ed. New York, NY: Holt, Rinehart & Winston; 1986.

Maccia ES, Maccia GS. The way of educational theorizing through models. In: Maccia ES, Maccia GS, Jewett RE, eds. *Construction of Educational Theory Models*. Washington, DC: Office of Education, US Dept of Health, Education, and Welfare, Cooperative Research Project No. 1632; 1963:30-45.

Pedhazur EJ, Schmelkin LP. *Measurement, Design, and Analysis: An Integrated Approach*. Hillsdale, NJ: Erlbaum; 1991.

Polit DF, Beck CT. *Nursing Research: Principles and Methods*. 7th ed. Philadelphia, Penn: Lippincott; 2003.

Rose MA, Shrader-Bogen CL, Korlath G, Priem J, Larson LR. Identifying patient symptoms after radiotherapy using a nurse-managed telephone interview. *Oncol Nurs Forum*. 1996;23:99-102.

Skinner BF. *Science and Human Behavior*. New York, NY: Free Press; 1953.

Wheeler JA. How come the quantum? In: Ferris T, ed. *The Best American Science Writing 2001*. New York, NY: HarperCollins; 2001:41-43.

ADDITIONAL READINGS

Maccia ES, Maccia GS. *Development of Educational Theory Derived from Three Educational Theory Models*. Washington, DC: Office of Education, US Dept of Health, Education, and Welfare, Project No. 5-0638; 1966.

Maccia ES, Maccia GS, Jewett RE, eds. *Construction of Educational Theory Models*. Washington, DC: Office of Education, US Dept of Health, Education, and Welfare, Cooperative Research Project No. 1632; 1963.

8

Statement Analysis

Preliminary Note: *Statement analysis may be used alone to examine hypotheses in a study or propositions in a theory. In addition, it provides a set of skills essential to theory analysis. Much of the examination of the logic of a theory is a result of a good solid analysis of each statement in the theory. So, even though you may not see formal articles about analyses of statements, it is a method you need to be very familiar with in order to do the work of science.*

DEFINITION AND DESCRIPTION

Examining relational statements to determine in what form they are presented and what relationship the concepts within those statements have to one another is the basic process of statement analysis. Statement analysis focuses on each concept within a statement, the relationships among concepts, and the role that the statement plays as a whole.

In Chapter 2 we listed two types of nonrelational statements used in theory. The first was what Reynolds (1971) called an *existence* statement that simply identifies a concept or an object and claims its existence. For example, we might say, "the phenomenon of a person's subjective feelings is termed the *affect*." The name of the concept "affect" is claimed to exist and is identified by a brief summary statement. Existence statements occur in theories to provide background and explanation prior to positing relationships.

A *definition* is the second type of nonrelational statement in a theory. A definition describes the characteristics of a concept. It may be a *theoretical* definition—one that is abstract and useful to the theory, but with no empirical referents named—or it may be an *operational* definition, in which the method of measurement is clearly spelled out. Leaving rods and cones out of it for now, let us assume that the concept of "color blindness" has a theoretical definition that implies visual inability to distinguish accurately between colors. The operational definition of color blindness, then, might include criteria such as which colors would be included in testing, how many times the test must be run, and how many "wrong" answers constitute failure before "color blindness" can be said to be present. Definitions are useful in theory because they provide the basis for clear communication between the theorist and the reader or user.

Relational statements are a bit more complex than either existence statements or definitions. Relational statements form the skeleton of a theory. Each statement describes some type of relationship among or between the concepts within it. When they occur singly they form the basis for research, or at least further reflection on the phenomena in question. When they occur in groups and are not interrelated, they provide the stimulus for thinking and exploring their possible linkages. If they occur in groups and are interrelated, they are called "theory" and form the basis for research programs.

Relational statements come in several forms or types. Suffice it to say that relational statements may be causal, probabilistic, concurrent, conditional, time-ordered, necessary, or sufficient (Hardy, 1974; Reynolds, 1971). Each of these forms will be discussed further later in this chapter.

PURPOSE AND USES

Statement analysis is a rigorous exercise. The purposes of statement analysis are (1) to classify statements as to form and (2) to examine the relationships among the concepts. The exercise provides a means of examining statements in an orderly way to determine if the statements are useful, informative, and logically correct.

Statement analysis provides a way of looking at and formalizing theoretical constructions that are already available in the literature or through research. Statement analysis is suited to situations in which one or more statements about a phenomenon exist but have not yet been organized into a theoretical system. The strategy is also useful in providing the theorist with information about the structure and function of the statements being considered. It is particularly useful because once the statement has been analyzed, any obvious deficiencies in it may be corrected or modified.

When a theorist is building a "new" theory, carefully examining the proposed relational statements using statement analysis will help the theorist "clean up" any problems before subjecting the new theory to criticism and scrutiny from the scholarly community.

STEPS IN STATEMENT ANALYSIS

The steps in statement analysis are not linear but iterative. The analyst will go back and forth through the various steps at odd intervals to be sure that things have been interpreted correctly. The more iterations achieved, the more likely a reasonable analysis will ensue. There are seven steps in statement analysis: (1) select the statement(s) to be analyzed; (2) simplify the statement; (3) classify the statement; (4) examine concepts within the statement for definition and validity; (5) specify relationships among concepts by type, sign, and symmetry; (6) examine the logic; and (7) determine testability.

Select the Statement

Selecting a statement to be analyzed involves some commitment to the idea behind the statement. Anyone attempting statement analysis should have clearly in mind what reason he or she has for doing so. Perhaps some doubt exists about the statement, or perhaps the idea is exciting, provoking examination of the content or structure for soundness before refuting or acting upon it in some way. In any case, the theorist should have the rationale for analysis clearly in mind before beginning.

One difficulty in selecting a statement is that some verbal or written theories suffer from a woeful lack of specificity in their relational statements. Theories, especially in the social and behavioral sciences, may be elaborately verbal (Blalock, 1969). On close inspection, however, it may prove quite difficult to isolate one single relational statement. It then becomes the task of the analyst to extract or construct simple relational statements from all the verbiage. This exercise requires very careful reading to accurately reflect the meaning the original theorist intended. Checking with colleagues or even the original theorist is often a big help when confronted by such a problem.

Finally, a statement selected for analysis must be relevant. That is, it is far better to select a prominent or major statement in a theory than to select an insignificant one. To tell the difference in major and minor statements, examine the statement's breadth. A major statement will yield more information to the analyst than a minor one will. In addition, if the major statement has validity, the likelihood increases that the minor one does too.

Simplify the Statement If Necessary

Simplifying a statement is needed only if one of two things occurs. The first is the problem of the elaborate verbal model that must be reduced to manageable statements. The second problem is complexity, which may occur in theories where one concept may be linked to several others simultaneously. When this happens, it simplifies analysis to break the concept linkages into several shorter, more manageable statements. Assume a statement could be diagrammed as the one in Figure 8–1. It is clear that the analyst might find the job much easier to handle if the formulation looked more like the one in Figure 8–2. The analyst now has four simple discrete relationships to examine instead of one set of complex relationships. It is also clear, however, that great care must be exercised when simplifying statements, or relationships may be overlooked or misconstrued.

Cooley's (1999) excellent analysis of Corbin and Strauss's (1991) trajectory theory of chronic illness management gives some nice examples of how to simplify complex propositions into manageable and analyzable statements. Corbin and Strauss's Proposition 1 stated, "Yet courses can be extended, kept stable, and their symptoms controlled through proper management" (p. 162). Cooley restated it to read: "Trajectory management can control symptoms, keep stable or extend the

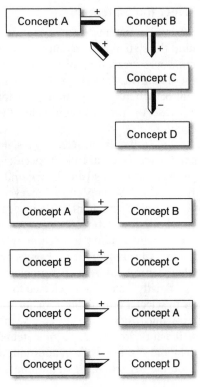

FIGURE 8–1 A complicated statement. See Figure 8–2 for simplification.

FIGURE 8–2 The statement in Figure 8–1 broken down into several shorter, more manageable statements.

trajectory" (p. 81). She used the placeholders *TM* for trajectory management and *T* for trajectory. She then diagrammed the statement as

$$TM \xrightarrow{+} T$$

Classify the Statement

As discussed, there are three basic classifications of statements: (1) existence statements, (2) definitions, and (3) relational statements.

Existence statements claim existence for concepts (Reynolds, 1971). The statement "That object is called a refrigerator" is an existence statement. Existence statements are not definitions and thus do not describe characteristics of the concept. They simply assert that something is so. Existence statements can be accurate or inaccurate. If the object in our example is really a dishwasher, then the statement is inaccurate. If the object in the statement corresponds to reality (it *is* a refrigerator) then the existence statement is accurate.

Definitions have three subforms—descriptive, stipulative, and operational (Hempel, 1966). A **descriptive** definition explains the accepted meaning for a term already in use. It explicates the term in other words that are already understood by the reader. It generally can be considered accurate. For example, a descriptive definition of "kitten" might read: "A kitten is the biological offspring of an adult female cat."

If the definition describes the term in such a way that it has a distinctive use assigned by the author and that may depart from the widely accepted use, then it is a **stipulative** definition. These definitions cannot be considered either accurate or inaccurate because they are specifically formulated *only* for use in the way the author of the theory has decreed. A stipulative definition of "kitten" might read: "For the purpose of this study, a kitten shall be defined as any healthy female offspring of a healthy female cat that is less than 8 weeks old." A stipulative definition is not the same as an operational definition.

An **operational** definition includes the specific means for measuring or testing each scientific term within it. An operational definition must be so precise that different scientists can use it repetitively and still obtain objective results. In our definition of "kitten," for instance, the operational definition might be: "For the purposes of this study, a kitten shall be any healthy offspring of a healthy female cat weighing between 4 and 12 ounces and no less than 3 days or more than 12 days old."

Relational statements specify relationships between concepts. Some relational statements may be so well supported empirically and logically that they function as laws or axioms within the theory. Others may be less well supported by data or logic and serve as propositions or empirical generalizations. Relational statements may also be hypotheses that are as yet unsupported by data even if they may appear reasonable and logical. Identifying the relational statements is very important when reaching step 5 in the statement analysis. It is that step in which the analyst specifies which *type* of relationship the statement exemplifies.

Examine the Concepts Within the Statement

Perhaps the easiest part of statement analysis is identifying the concepts within the statement to be analyzed. Scan the statement for the major ideas expressed within it. The names, or terms, for these ideas are the pertinent concepts.

There are three actions involved in examining the concepts once they are identified. The first is to determine the definitions of the terms that reflect the concepts. The definition should reflect all the defining attributes of the concept so that everyone who reads the theory will know precisely how the theorist intends the term to be used. (For a discussion of determining defining attributes for a concept, see Chapter 5.) If the concept is not adequately defined, can its meaning be determined from the context of the theoretical formulation? If so, the analyst should use this material to help formulate additions to the definition that will aid the analysis and even, perhaps, help refine the theory. If not, then the analyst must simply state that the concepts are inadequately defined for the purpose of analysis.

Determining if the concepts *as they are defined* are theoretically valid is the second step in the examination of concepts in a statement. The analyst attempts to determine whether the concepts, as they are defined, accurately reflect the general semantic usage for that concept. This process involves a brief review of the relevant literature concerning the concept being considered. If the concept is being used in the same ways as it has previously been used in the literature and the definition reflects it, the concept may be considered valid. When the theorist has conducted a careful concept analysis, the concept is considered valid even if it does not reflect the relevant literature but goes beyond traditional usage. In fact, the validity of the concept may be more certain *after* analysis than a concept defined by tradition alone.

Finally, determine if the concepts, *as they are defined,* are used consistently throughout the discussions related to the formation of the statement. Occasionally, an author will subtly change the meaning of a concept in an attempt to make the meaning clear or will define the concept clearly and then change it slightly to reflect the measuring instrument's definition. The analyst should be aware of this possibility and make a note of any changes that may occur.

Specify Relationships by Type, Sign, and Symmetry

Assessment of a relational statement for type, sign, and symmetry is to determine its function within the theory. In the interest of clarity and simplicity, we assume that all relational statements are linear until proven otherwise. (Statement analysis can often provide the clue to curvilinear relationships. If you can't classify a statement or determine its sign, it may express a nonlinear relationship.)

Type   Several types of relational statements may occur. These are causal, probabilistic, concurrent, conditional, time-ordered, necessary, and sufficient (Hardy, 1974). We will consider each type briefly giving examples of each.

A **causal** statement is one in which the first concept is said to be the "cause" of the other. Causal statements are often deduced from laws. Therefore, there are very few causal statements in the social and behavioral sciences primarily because they encompass so many intervening variables that may influence causation. Causality is easier to demonstrate in the physical sciences. For example, the statement "Raising the temperature of a gas held under constant pressure will increase its volume" is a causal statement. It asserts that some event (raising the temperature of a gas under constant pressure) causes another event (increased gas volume). This is the simplest form of causal statement, although there are more complex ones involving several causal factors for one phenomenon. Causal statements are difficult to find in health and social sciences, especially in beginning attempts at theory construction, because the caused outcome must *always* happen if the causal event or events occur.

It is often helpful to use symbols, or placeholders, for the concepts in statements to avoid becoming confused by the content of the concepts during analysis. Using the symbols G_p for gas under pressure, T for temperature, and GV for gas volume, the analyst could diagram the previous causal statement thus

$$\text{If } \uparrow T \rightarrow G_p, \text{ then always } \uparrow GV.$$

If the event (GV) always occurs, it can be labeled a causal statement.

A statement is called **probabilistic** if the event occurs some of the time or most of the time, but not *all* of the time. Probabilistic statements are usually derived from statistical data. They assert that if one event occurs, the second event probably will also. An excellent example of a probabilistic statement is that cigarette smoking (*CS*) is highly likely to lead to lung cancer (*LC*). There is no direct causality in this statement because everyone who smokes does not develop lung cancer. But the *probability* of developing lung cancer is increased significantly in the presence of cigarette smoking. This probabilistic relationship, if diagrammed, might look like this:

$$\text{If } CS \rightarrow \text{then probably } LC.$$

When a statement asserts that if event A occurs, event B also occurs, it is asserting that the relationship between the concepts is **concurrent**. There may or may not be any causation between the two events—they simply exist together. An example of this kind of statement might be: "A low level of educational preparation and a low income often occur together." The statement does not infer that lack of education *causes* poverty. Another example of concurrence can be found in Muhlenkamp and Parsons's classic study of nurses (1972) and is confirmed in Kaiser and Bickle's study (1980). These authors found that nurses have personality characteristics that are highly feminine rather than masculine. This is a good example of a concurrent statement. It simply asserts that nurses (*N*) and feminine personality (*FP*) characteristics occur together. It makes no other claim. A diagram of this statement would be

$$\text{If } N, \text{ also } FP.$$

Sometimes a relationship between two concepts occurs only in the presence of a third concept. This type of statement is a **conditional** statement. A good example of a conditional statement is one found in a series of studies by Acton, Irvin, Jensen, Hopkins, and Miller (1997) on the mediating effects of self-care resources. In their studies they found that the relationship between high levels of stress (*HS*) and diminished well-being (*DMB*) was improved when subjects had higher levels of social support (*SS*), self-worth (*SW*), and hope (*H*). This can be simplistically diagrammed as

$$\text{If } HS, \text{ then } DMB, \text{ but not in presence of } SS, SW, \text{ and } H.$$

Time-ordered statements are those that indicate that some amount of time intervenes between the first concept or event and the second. An example of a time-ordered statement is the classic one indicating that when a person experiences numerous stressful life events (*SLE*) within a year the likelihood of that person becoming ill (*I*) is quite high (Erickson, Tomlin, & Swain, 1990; Holmes & Rahe, 1968; Rahe, 1972). This relationship is time-ordered because time passes between the first episodes of stress and the resultant illness. This statement can be diagrammed like this:

If *SLE*, then later *I*.

A statement that indicates that one and only one concept or event can lead to the second concept or event reflects a **necessary** relationship. Necessary relationships function very much as differential diagnoses do in medicine. That is, a patient can be positively said to have cancer, for instance, if and only if there is a pathologist's report of malignant cells on biopsy. In the same way, relationships among concepts may occur only under certain conditions. An example from nursing might be a statement relating to stress and adaptation. Roy's (1976), Neuman's (1980), and Erickson and colleagues' (1990) models of nursing have all stated that adaptation (*A*) occurs as a response to stressors (*S*). Stressors then become *necessary* before adaptation can occur. The diagram would look like this:

If and only if *S*, then *A*.

Statements in which the first concept or event and the second concept or event are related, regardless of anything else, demonstrate **sufficient** relationships. Using the stressor–adaptation idea above, we can see that if stressors occur then adaptation will begin in the person whether or not she or he wills it and whether or not someone intervenes. In other words, the presence of the first concept guarantees the presence of the second concept. A sufficient relationship could be diagrammed this way:

If *S*, then *A*, regardless of anything else.

When first introduced to statement analysis, some students mistakenly believe that a statement can be only one type at a time. This is clearly not the case. For instance, most relational statements are probabilistic *in addition* to being conditional or concurrent or time-ordered and so on.

Sign   Signs generally fall into one of three categories: positive, negative, or unknown (Mullins, 1971; Reynolds, 1971). The rule of thumb is that if the concepts vary in the same direction, that is, as one increases or decreases so does the other, then the relationship is positive. If one concept increases while the other decreases, the relationship is said to be negative. If you have no information about the way the concepts vary, the relationship is unknown. Below are three probabilistic statements and one statement inferred from the first three with their relationships drawn to help you see how this is done:

When members of a group become anxious (*A*), hostility (*H*) increases.

$$A \xrightarrow{+} H$$

Hostility is related to a decrease in group cohesiveness (GC).

$$H \xrightarrow{-} GC$$

Creativity (C) decreases as anxiety increases in groups.

$$A \xrightarrow{-} C$$

Inferred: Anxiety has a negative impact on group cohesiveness.

$$A \xrightarrow{-} GC$$

This inferred statement was derived logically from the first two statements. Because both A and GC are related to H, they are therefore related to each other.

What we cannot tell from these four statements is what effect creativity and group cohesiveness have on each other. So that might look like this:

$$C \xrightarrow{?} GC$$

Symmetry   So far, all our examples have been asymmetrical, that is, one-direction relationships. In asymmetrical statements, the relationship goes from only one concept to the next but is never reciprocated. There are many examples of asymmetrical relationships in our discussions. One example is the statement above that anxiety is negatively related to group cohesiveness. But, relationships can be symmetrical as well (Blalock, 1969) where each concept affects the other. An example of a symmetrical statement might be one from research done by one of us on maternal attachment behaviors (Avant, 1981). High attachment scores (At) were associated with low anxiety (Ax) scores and high anxiety scores were associated with low attachment scores in primiparous women. This relationship can be diagrammed like this:

$$At \xleftrightarrow{-} Ax$$

Examine the Logic

Origin, reasonableness, and adequacy are the criteria for examining the logic of relationships. When examining the origin of a statement, ask yourself whether the statement is constructed deductively, that is from a more general law, or inductively, from observation or available data. If the statement is deductive in origin, its logic should be adequate because a conclusion in a deductive argument cannot be false if the premises are true. If the statement is inductive, its logic cannot be judged except by the amount of empirical support it has and by comparison to existing knowledge (Hempel, 1966). If it has strong support in both empirical testing and in agreement with existing literature, its logic is probably adequate. The logic can also be determined by examining the relationships of the concepts to each other. If the relationship cannot be classified by type, sign, or symmetry there may be a logical flaw.

Determining the reasonableness of a statement also uses comparison to existing knowledge. Simply ask if this statement seems reasonable given what you already know on the subject. If it makes sense in the light of existing knowledge, it is reasonable.

Determining adequacy of a single statement is more difficult than determining adequacy of a theory because we cannot construct matrices or models to demonstrate where logical gaps may occur. It is possible, however, to draw a simple diagram as we have done in the previous section labeling the concepts by letters or numbers and determining types and signs that are relevant. If you are unable to do any one of the three, there is some flaw in the statement.

Determine Testability

In this final step of the analysis, determine whether or not there are operational measures that can be used in the real world to obtain data that will support or refute the statement being analyzed. It is at this point that the analyst will run up against the situation Hempel calls "testability-in-principle." Basically, this is a statement that *could* be tested empirically if the tools were available to measure the concepts; but they are not available (Hempel, 1966). He considers these statements just as useful in theory construction as the empirically testable statements. We feel that the criterion of testability can be met if a statement is either testable-in-principle or actually testable because so many concepts in nursing may lack the instruments to measure them. This is not to imply, however, that all statements are therefore testable.

In order for a statement to meet the criterion of testability it must render some test implications. That is, you should be able to say: "If I tested this under the specified conditions, then the outcome hypothesized should actually happen." A relatively "new" statement might render fewer testable ideas than one that has more age and support, but if it is testable at all, it meets the criterion. Any statement that cannot produce one testable idea or that is constructed in such a way that the concepts have vague meanings, cannot meet the criterion of testability until modified.

ADVANTAGES AND LIMITATIONS

The primary advantage of statement analysis is that it provides a systematic way of examining the relationships among concepts. In addition, it assists the theorist in examining the structure and function of statements. Statement analysis is also a fundamental skill necessary for theory analysis. But perhaps the most important function of statement analysis occurs when the theorist is thinking carefully and systematically about the linkages between concepts. He or she may discover other linkages or relationships that are important to the final theoretical formulations during that thinking time. In just such analysis situations many scientists have "happened on to" significant theoretical ideas.

Analyzing just *one* statement may be a limitation of statement analysis, especially if it is part of a theoretical whole. Removing the statement from its context can often result in loss of valuable information, and the analysis is hindered. In addition, determining the logic of a statement is often more difficult when it is removed from the theory. The final limitation of the statement analysis process is that it does take a little time and it is rigorous. This is a limitation only as it applies to the theorist, however; this very intense and time-consuming effort ultimately proves very valuable in assessing statements.

UTILIZING THE RESULTS OF STATEMENT ANALYSIS

Statement analysis results in formalized statements with their underlying structures and functions made explicit. But what does a theorist do with the resulting information? It can be used in a variety of ways in education, practice, research, and theory development.

Analyzed statements can be used as springboards for discussion in the classroom. Discussions may include ideas about which concepts were clear, which ones were related to each other, and how, or what, inconsistencies were discovered. The amount of empirical evidence for or against the statement can provide the basis for designing classroom activities such as proposals for research studies to produce either more evidence in support of the statement or more evidence to falsify it. The amount of empirical evidence could also be used to launch a discussion about the efficacy of the statement to guide clinical practice.

Another possible use for statement analysis in education would be having a faculty interest group discuss the issues raised from analyzing several similar statements or several statements about the same selected topic. This discussion could lead to curriculum changes or to faculty research projects. A series of faculty discussions and analyses had just such a result in the development of the theory of unpleasant symptoms (Lenz, Pugh, Milligan, Gift, & Suppe, 1997; Lenz, Suppe, Gift, Pugh, & Milligan, 1995).

Statement analysis can guide clinicians in the judicious use of research findings. Knowing whether or not a statement is associational, causal, or time-ordered can inform decisions about when to use the statement and under what conditions. Certain nursing diagnoses may be considered or certain nursing interventions or outcomes chosen as a result of a statement analysis not previously available to the nurse. In addition, faced with the choice of two potential interventions, the nurse using results from a statement analysis would know which one has the most empirical support, thus leading to a more educated decision.

Statement analysis allows the researcher or theorist to identify the problems in a statement and to take the appropriate next step. Concepts may need clarifying. Inconsistencies, unclear definitions, and gaps in knowledge can become apparent. Together, these clarifications provide direction for planning concept analyses, reformulating ideas, or proposing new hypotheses to test. Connell, Shaw, Holmes, and Foster's (2001) article on family participation in Alzheimer's research offers an excellent example of how statement analysis can be useful in research and practice.

If the analysis has demonstrated that the statement is sound, the theorist can begin to look for other concepts and linkages to add to what is already known. This is how theories are built—one step at a time.

SUMMARY

Statement analysis is a process of systematically examining the relationships among concepts. There are seven steps involved: selecting the statement; simplifying it if necessary; classifying it; examining the concepts for definition and validity; specifying relationships by type, sign, and symmetry; examining the logic; and determining the testability.

Once a statement has been analyzed, any deficiencies in the statement are clear and may be corrected. Furthermore, the process of thinking aloud, discussions, and written assessments often generate additional ideas and statements, either by deduction or by serendipity, that are valuable additions to future theoretical formulations.

PRACTICE EXERCISES

Below are several statements from a study of faculty attitudes (Ruiz, 1981).

A. Classify each statement as either
   a. Relational statement
   b. Descriptive definition
   c. Stipulative definition
   d. Operational definition
      1. Ethnocentrism means ethnic narrow-mindedness.
      2. Dogmatism shall be defined as close-mindedness.
      3. Intolerance of ambiguity and dogmatism are the two factors underlying ethnocentrism for this study.
      4. Faculty who are highly dogmatic view patients with different ethnocultural backgrounds as annoying and superstitious.
      5. Faculty who have high ethnocentrism scores have negative attitudes toward culturally different patients.
B. Using statement 4, simplify it into two statements and diagram them.
C. Using statements 4 and 5, examine the concepts and specify the relationships by type, sign, and symmetry. Determine the logic and testability of each.

Answers

A. 1. b; 2. c; 3. d; 4. a; 5. a
B. 1. Dogmatic faculty (*DF*) view patients with differing ethnocultural (*DEB*) backgrounds as annoying (*A*):

If *DF*, then *A*, but only if *DEB*.

2. Dogmatic faculty (*DF*) view patients with differing ethnocultural backgrounds (*DEB*) as superstitious (*S*):

   If *DF*, then *S*, but only if *DEB*.

C. Statement 4 can be diagrammed as *DF* $\overset{-}{\rightarrow}$ *A* and *S*, but only if *DEB*.

   Statement 5 can be diagrammed as ethnocentric faculty (*EF*) $\overset{-}{\rightarrow}$ attitudes toward culturally different patients (*ACDP*) or *EF* $\overset{-}{\rightarrow}$ *ACDP*.

Both statements 4 and 5 are probabilistic because they are drawn from statistical data. Statement 4, as it is diagrammed in Practice Exercise B, is conditional as well. Both statements are asymmetrical. The signs are negative because less dogmatic faculty had more positive views of ethnocentric patients.

Some of the concepts from statements 4 and 5, such as "patient," "faculty," "ethnocultural background," "annoying," and "superstitious," are undefined. If these concepts were intended to be used in their common language meanings, the author should state that clearly. Otherwise, each should be defined. The two concepts that were defined, "ethnocentrism" and "dogmatism," are given only in vague, equally undefined terms in this exercise. (They were operationally defined in the actual study.) The concept of "intolerance of ambiguity" is not defined but is used as part of an operational definition. This is clearly to be avoided. None of the concept definitions are unambiguous.

The statements are logical. They are testable only if better concept definitions are constructed so that operational measures can be found for them. It can be said that the concepts are measurable or the statement testable only when there are careful operational definitions that reflect the theoretical definitions.

REFERENCES

Acton GJ, Irvin BL, Jensen BA, Hopkins BA, Miller EW. Explicating middle-range theory through methodological diversity. *Adv Nurs Sci.* 1997;19(3):78-85.

Avant K. Anxiety as a potential factor affecting maternal attachment. *J Obstet Gynecol Neonatal Nurs.* 1981;10(6):416-420.

Blalock H Jr. *Theory Construction: From Verbal to Mathematical Formulations.* Englewood Cliffs, NJ: Prentice Hall; 1969.

Connell CM, Shaw BA, Holmes SB, Foster NL. Caregiver's attitudes toward their family members' participation in Alzheimer disease research: implications for recruitment and retention. *Alzheimer Dis Assoc Disord.* 2001;15(3):137-145.

Cooley ME. Analysis and evaluation of the trajectory of chronic illness management. *Scholar Inquiry Nurs Pract.* 1999;13(2):75-95.

Corbin JM, Strauss A. A nursing model for chronic illness management based upon the trajectory framework. *Scholar Inquiry Nurs Pract.* 1991;5:155-174.

Erickson HC, Tomlin E, Swain MA. *Modeling and Role-Modeling: A Theory and Paradigm for Nursing.* Lexington, SC: Pine Press; 1990.

Hardy M. Theories: components, development, and evaluation. *Nurs Res.* 1974;23:100-107.

Hempel C. *Philosophy of Natural Science.* Englewood Cliffs, NJ: Prentice Hall; 1966.

Holmes R, Rahe R. The social readjustment rating scale. *J Psychosom Res.* 1968;11:213-218.

Kaiser J, Bickle I. Attitude change as a motivational factor in producing behavior change related to implementing primary nursing. *Nurs Res.* 1980;19(5):290-300.

Lenz ER, Pugh LC, Milligan RA, Gift AG, Suppe F. The middle-range theory of unpleasant symptoms: an update. *Adv Nurs Sci.* 1997;19(3):14-27.

Lenz ER, Suppe F, Gift AG, Pugh LC, Milligan RA. Collaborative development of middle-range nursing theories: toward a theory of unpleasant symptoms. *Adv Nurs Sci.* 1995; 17(3):1-13.

Muhlenkamp A, Parsons J. Characteristics of nurses: an overview of recent research published in a nursing research periodical. *J Vocational Behav.* 1972;2:261-273.

Mullins N. *The Art of Theory: Construction and Use.* New York, NY: Harper & Row; 1971.

Neuman B. The Betty Neuman health-care systems model. In: Riehl J P, Roy C, eds. *Conceptual Models for Nursing Practice.* 2nd ed. New York, NY: Appleton-Century-Crofts; 1980.

Rahe R. Subject's recent life changes and their near future illness susceptibility. *Adv Psychosom Med.* 1972;8:2-19.

Reynolds P. *A Primer in Theory Construction.* Indianapolis, Ind: Bobbs-Merrill; 1971.

Roy C. *Introduction to Nursing: An Adaptation Model.* Englewood Cliffs, NJ: Prentice Hall; 1976.

Ruiz M. Open-closed mindedness, intolerance of ambiguity and nursing faculty attitudes toward culturally different patients. *Nurs Res.* 1981;30(3):177-181.

ADDITIONAL READINGS

Greenwood D. *The Nature of Science and Other Essays.* New York, NY: Philosophical Library; 1959.

Hage J. *Techniques and Problems of Theory Construction in Sociology.* New York, NY: Wiley; 1972.

Lerner D, ed. *Parts and Wholes.* New York, NY: Free Press of Glencoe; 1963.

Zetterberg HL. *On Theory and Verification in Sociology.* 3rd ed. New York, NY: Bedminster Press; 1965.

PART IV

Theory Development

Theory development is greatly needed in nursing, especially the middle-range theory that bridges the gap between the metaparadigm concepts and practice. However, "good" theory development takes time and work. It is a very sophisticated and complex level of effort because the theorist must deal with concepts, statements, linkages, and definitions all at the same time. Using the strategies in the next three chapters should help the theorist begin appropriate level theory development.

Theory development is needed when there are concepts or even relational statements about the theorist's area of interest, but no way to link them together. In this case, the most useful strategies might be theory synthesis (Chapter 9) or theory derivation (Chapter 10). Theory development may also be needed when there is already theory on the topic of interest. Theory analysis (Chapter 11) would provide the theorist a means of examining the theory to determine its strengths and weaknesses. Once the strengths and weaknesses are known, then further development or testing can be done.

Finally, theory development might be needed when there is a body of literature, but it has been unfruitful in suggesting hypotheses for testing, or the data it contains are dated or outmoded. In this case any one of the three strategies might be helpful. Theory analysis could indicate deficits and inconsistencies in the current theories. Theory synthesis could provide a means of combining concepts and statements in a new way that could offer insights and provide new hypotheses. Theory derivation could provide concepts or a new structure for the concepts that might produce an interesting new unifying idea about the phenomenon of interest.

Deciding which strategy will be most useful depends on asking questions about the level of theory development, the type of literature available on the topic, and the quality and completeness of the literature. Theory development is the most challenging pursuit of the scientist, but it is also the most creative and the most satisfying.

9

Theory Synthesis

Preliminary Note: *The strategy of theory synthesis exemplifies the process of transforming practice-related research about phenomena of interest into an integrated whole. Such an integrated whole allows the theorist to bring bits and pieces of knowledge together in a more useful and coherent form. Because some readers may find it daunting to think of synthesizing a theory, it is probably more useful to think first of this strategy as a means for making sense of a jumble of facts, or bringing order to the process of a specific nursing intervention. Later, after the work is completed, dialogue and feedback from colleagues can help the aspiring theory builder determine how best to depict the work to the larger nursing community.*

DEFINITION AND DESCRIPTION

The aim of theory synthesis is construction of a theory, an interrelated system of ideas, from empirical evidence. In this strategy a theorist pulls together available information about a phenomenon. Concepts and statements are organized into a network or whole, a synthesized theory. Theory synthesis involves three steps or phases: (1) specifying focal concepts to serve as anchors for the synthesized theory, (2) reviewing the literature to identify factors related to the focal concepts and to specify the nature of relationships, and (3) organizing concepts and statements into an integrated and efficient representation of the phenomena of interest.

Theory synthesis results in a more complex representation of phenomena than either concept or statement synthesis. This is true for several reasons. In contrast to concepts, which serve to highlight phenomena of interest, theories demonstrate the connections among concepts. Further, theories simultaneously embrace more aspects of phenomena and integrate them more thoroughly than statements. Although a statement may link only two or three concepts together (Figure 9–1a), a theory may connect a number of concepts to each other and also specify complex direct and indirect linkages among concepts (Figure 9–1b). Theories offer still other benefits. A theory that is well designed moves beyond existing knowledge by pointing the way to new and surprising discoveries (Causey, 1969; Hempel, 1966, pp. 70–84).

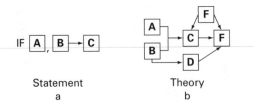

Statement
a

Theory
b

FIGURE 9–1 Example of complexity of linkages in statement (a) versus theory (b).

Theories that are synthesized may be presented in more than one way. When the relationships within and among statements are depicted in graphic form, this constitutes a *model* of the phenomenon (see Chapter 2 on the terminology of theory construction). In this chapter we will use the terms *theory* and *theoretical model* interchangeably because it is often quite useful to represent beginning theories in both graphic (model) and linguistic (theory) form. Theorists often move back and forth between expressing theories in written sentences and visual devices, such as diagrams, during theory construction. In the final stages of theory building and refinement, theories may also be expressed in mathematical form (Blalock, 1969). Here, given that this is an introductory book on theory construction, we will limit ourselves to linguistic and graphic expressions of theory.

Like other synthesis strategies, theory synthesis builds on a base of empirical evidence. In theory synthesis, a theorist may combine information from various sources during theory building: qualitative and quantitative observations, available data banks, and published research findings. In utilizing qualitative and statistical information in theory synthesis, it is helpful to first translate them into relational statements (see Chapter 6 on statement synthesis). Because a theorist can use a variety of sources of data in theory synthesis, we will not present distinct methods for each source. Rather, we will attend to each source of data within an overall strategy for theory synthesis. A theorist may utilize evidence from each of these sources in the construction of a particular model. In theory synthesis the source of data is less important than the salience of the evidence to the phenomenon represented by the model.

Readers should keep in mind that a synthesized theory is limited in its generalizability or external validity by the extent and quality of evidence upon which it is based. Theoretical models drawn from a limited number of sources normally will be more restricted in focus and less generalizable than ones based on multiple and diverse sources. Synthesis strategies are more "grounded" in reality, however, than other strategies such as derivation because they are based on real data. Synthesized theories, like synthesized statements, require testing or cross-validating to reaffirm their empirical validity.

A working knowledge of statistical concepts is a valuable tool in theory synthesis that draws on quantitative data. Knowledge of statistics enables a theorist to directly utilize statistical information to which he or she has access in theory construction. Further, theorists who are conversant in statistics are better able to critically evaluate the accuracy of statements based on others' statistical findings. Nevertheless, because our focus in this chapter is on the process of theory synthesis, we will keep our use of statistical information to a minimum.

Because it is probably easiest to get a grasp on how theory synthesis works by demonstrating the process, we provide the following illustration. We draw on a literature review and qualitative study done by Ward (2002) on the topic of transformational leadership, a visionary style of leadership characterized by qualities such as power sharing that are conducive to organizational development. Our illustration is not intended as a comprehensive presentation on this topic. Readers who find the topic of particular interest are referred to Ward's original article for more complete details. (*Note:* We have identified factors related to transformational leadership by assigning an alphabetical letter [A, B, etc.] to it. These letters are also included in the model constructed from Ward's literature review [Figure 9–2] so that readers may trace the translation made from linguistic to graphic representation of the findings.)

From Ward's article we extracted the following antecedents of transformational leadership. Included among these antecedents are having a personal support system *(A)*, having certain personal characteristics such as self-confidence *(B)*, and pursuit of a career pathway *(C)*. Studies also indicated that increased worker retention *(D)*, decreased absenteeism *(E)*, and increased job satisfaction *(F)* are among organizational outcomes of transformational leadership *(G)*. Because Ward does not mention if errors *(H)* are reduced by transformational leadership, we cannot make a conclusion about relationships to this important organizational outcome. Having identified a series of relationships pertinent to transformational leadership, we then constructed a diagram, Figure 9–2, to represent the relationships as an interrelated network of ideas. In constructing Figure 9–2, the symbols +, ?, and − were used to designate, respectively, factors with positive, unknown, and negative relationships to transformational leadership. For simplicity, we treated the relationships as unidirectional and causal in our illustration. (See Chapter 6 for further discussion of the concepts of directionality and causality.)

Our example of a model of transformational leadership was based in most cases on reported research findings. Had we access to a data bank on transformational leadership we might have generated further information pertinent to the

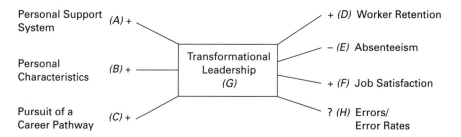

FIGURE 9–2 Model of transformational leadership. (For more complete information, see Ward, 2002.)

model. Suppose we had done this and found that transformational leadership was correlated ($r = .50$) with positive lifestyle changes in employees, such as smoking reduction. We then would have added changes in lifestyle to the model as an outcome of transformational leadership. Statistical information translated into a statement of relationship may be entered into a theoretical model in the same way as relationships gleaned from the literature. Similarly, findings from qualitative research also may be added to the model.

PURPOSE AND USES

The aim of theory synthesis is to represent a phenomenon through an interrelated set of concepts and statements. Three specific aims for theory synthesis include the following:

1. To represent the factors that precede or influence a particular event, such as factors that lead women to be screened for osteoporosis, or to leave abusive relationships.
2. To represent effects that occur after some event, such as outcomes following nursing interventions with rural elders.
3. To put related, but discrete scientific information into a more theoretically organized form, such as modeling the factors that lead immigrant groups to adopt acculturated dietary practices.

Using theory synthesis for the third purpose involves organizing relational statements into a system and collapsing factors or variables that resemble each other into larger summary concepts. Conducting theory synthesis for this last purpose is less concerned with depicting relationships about a phenomenon than focusing on improving the overall form and quality with which a theory is expressed. In contrast, the first purpose may be especially directed to predicting and perhaps modifying some clinical event. The second is similarly helpful in predicting and ameliorating effects that are undesired consequences of a clinical phenomenon. The varied purposes of theory synthesis are equally valid. The specific purpose for which a theorist engages in theory synthesis will depend on the interests of the theorist and the use envisioned for the synthesized theory.

The type and amount of available evidence influences which of the three specific aims of theory synthesis will be most feasible in any given situation. For example, if only minimal information is available about the effects of some phenomenon, but a great deal is known about its antecedents or determinants, a theorist's efforts may be more profitably spent on theory synthesis related to antecedents. Generally, there must be research evidence available about relationships among at least three factors for theory synthesis to be possible. If this is not the case, the theorist should consider another strategy, for example, statement synthesis or theory derivation. The richer the pool of research information available to the theorist, the greater the complexity and precision possible in a synthesized theory.

Theory synthesis may be used in a wide variety of scientific and practical situations. It may be used to produce a compact graphic representation of research findings on a topic of interest. Literature reviews about multiple and complex relationships may be made less tedious and more informative through theory synthesis. Particularly where a graphic display of a synthesized theory is made, complex relations may be communicated more effectively than through traditional written reviews. This particular use of theory synthesis is relevant in teaching complex content about a clinical topic, applying research to the design of clinical interventions, and developing a theoretical framework for a research project.

Theory synthesis requires that a theorist systematically assess relationships among factors pertinent to a topic of interest. The process aids in highlighting areas in need of further research as the theorist methodically identifies relationships among variables; notes the directionality of the relationships; specifies whether the relationship is positive, negative, neutral, or unknown; and notes the quality and amount of evidence in support of the relationship. This information can be helpful in locating specific questions in need of further investigation.

PROCEDURES FOR THEORY SYNTHESIS

A common set of procedures comprises theory synthesis regardless of purpose. Although we outline the procedures as a set of steps or phases, their order is not absolute nor will a theorist necessarily devote comparable time to each.

Specify Focal Concepts

A theorist begins theory synthesis by marking off a topic of interest. The theorist may do this by specifying (a) *one focal concept* or variable, such as transformational leadership, or (b) a *framework* of several focal concepts. In the former case, the theorist moves out from the focal concept, for example, transformational leadership, to other concepts or variables related to it. In the latter case, the theorist is concerned with a framework of focal concepts and how they may be interrelated. For example, the relationship of various teacher attitudes and behaviors to various nursing student attitudes and behaviors constitutes a framework of focal concepts for beginning theory synthesis. Finally, if the focal concept(s) is expressed by several terms at more than one level of abstraction, a higher-order concept(s) should be selected to capture those equivalent terms. (See Chapter 6.)

Identify Related Factors and Relationships

Guided by a single focal concept or a framework of concepts, a careful search and review of the literature is done next. During the review, note is taken of variables related to the focal concept or framework of concepts. Relationships identified are systematically recorded indicating, where possible, whether they are bi- or unidirectional; positive, neutral, negative, or unknown; and weak, ambiguous, or strong in supporting evidence. Locating relationships in research may be facilitated by finding comprehensive and thorough review articles already written. If recent reviews on the focal concepts are not available, a thorough search of the literature is in order. Relationship statements are not located in one uniform place in research articles and reports. They may occur in the abstract, literature review, hypotheses, results, or discussion of a study. In a structured abstract, however, key relationships will be stated as conclusions. If the results of a study are not summarized in statement form, a theorist may have to trace a statement from the hypothesis section through the results section in order to determine if it was supported by actual findings of the study. This second step or phase may also be expanded to include other than literary sources of statements and concepts; for example, qualitative or quantitative observations made by the theorist may be translated into relational statements and then treated as any other statement in theory synthesis. (Readers may find Chapter 6 on statement synthesis helpful in clarifying and combining statements.)

Construct an Integrated Representation

Finally, when a theorist has collected a fairly representative listing of relational statements pertinent to one or more focal concepts, these may then be organized in terms of the overall pattern of relationships among variables. Diagrams are particularly helpful in expressing relationships among concepts and constitute the major device a theorist may use at this step to organize material. Readers will recall that in our illustration variables were organized into those that appeared to be antecedents of transformational leadership and those that appeared to be outcomes of it (see Figure 9–2). For each topic of interest a theorist must determine what is a reasonable basis for organizing statements.

Several mechanisms can facilitate organizing concepts into suitable networks of ideas. One such mechanism is to collapse several highly similar variables into a more comprehensive summary concept for use in the theory. For example, smiling, kissing, and cuddling a baby might all be amalgamated into a summary concept of parental attachment behavior. Similarly, return to work, normal blood sugar, and adherence to a prescribed diet may be collapsed under the concept of adaptation to chronic disease. Collapsing discrete variables into summary variables can make a theory more easily understood by reducing needless complexity. A more parsimonious theory will also be achieved by this method. Readers may find Chapter 3 on concept synthesis helpful in constructing summary concepts.

Another mechanism is organizing statements into what Zetterberg (1965) called an "inventory of determinants" or an "inventory of results." These refer respectively to the cataloging of antecedents and effects of a focal concept or variable. Structurally, these two types of inventories are quite similar. They differ only in whether the focal concept is viewed as an outcome of certain variables or a determinant of them (Figure 9–3). Organizing statements into inventories of determinants and results is often helpful where a theorist is dealing with only one focal concept or variable. This was the mechanism that we used for transformational leadership.

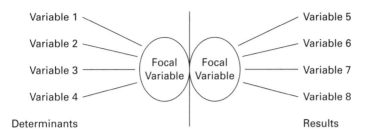

FIGURE 9–3   Inventories of determinants and results.

Yet another mechanism is Blalock's (1969) notion of theoretical "blocks." With this approach, variables that are more proximally related are organized together into a "block" and their interrelationships specified. Each block of variables is then related to more distally related variables in other blocks (Figure 9–4). Organizing variables and relationships into theoretical blocks is especially relevant if a theorist is constructing a "megamodel" comprised of several "minimodels."

The mechanisms cited above are only suggestions. A theorist must follow the evolving understanding that comes from carefully considering the existing literature and evidence in deciding how best to depict the phenomena of interest. Finally, an additional aid now available to theorists is computer software, such as arcs©, which can be used to manage and link variables derived from literature (see Additional Readings at the end of this chapter).

To reiterate our point at the beginning of this section, the three steps or phases of theory synthesis may be varied or expanded as needed. For example, conducting the literature review first may be necessary to help theorists clarify the focal concepts of greatest interest to them. In turn, organizing the concepts into an integrated network may be embellished by organizing concepts and relational statements in diagrams and then further coding them as to the extent of research support (*** = high support, * = low support, ? = conflicting support).

ILLUSTRATIONS OF THEORY SYNTHESIS

A classic and exemplary illustration of the process of theory synthesis is the model of adherence among hypertensive patients presented by Caplan, Robinson, French, Caldwell, and Shinn (1976). Caplan et al. began model construction by specifying the major dependent variables of interest: adherence and the lowering of blood pressure. They then worked backward to identify predictors or determinants of these focal variables. In constructing the model they expressed the hope that it would "serve as a heuristic aid in thinking about determinants of adherence" (p. 22). Below are key statements, largely paraphrased for brevity, that culminated in the Caplan et al. model.

Evidence supports relationships between maintaining blood pressure in normal limits and the goal of longevity, if not a long satisfying life (relationship A). Adherence to medical regimens that involve taking medications is an effective means of

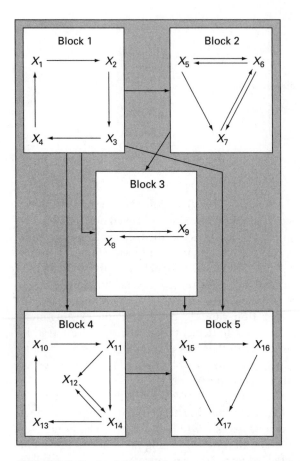

FIGURE 9–4 Variables and statements organized into theoretical blocks. *Source: Theory Construction: From Verbal to Mathematical Formulations* by Blalock, Hubert M., © 1969. Reprinted by permission of Pearson Education, Inc., Upper Saddle River, NJ.

controlling high blood pressure (relationship *B*). In attaining adherence, setting specific subgoals is important in goal attainment, and "rewards need to be anticipated, or explicitly identified in advance before the person begins to strive toward the goal" (Caplan et al., p. 26) to meet the desired level of adherence (relationship *D*). Further, patients' actual adherent behaviors "serve as a feedback mechanism helping them set new goals based on past accomplishments" (relationship *D*; p. 30). Accomplishment enhances patients' perceived competence to adhere (relationship *E*). Perceived competence to adhere leads to further adherence behavior (relationship *C*).

Caplan and Colleagues (1976) represented these relational statements in the graphic form shown in Figure 9–5. In this figure, letters are used to connect relational statements in linguistic form with their translation into graphic form. Of

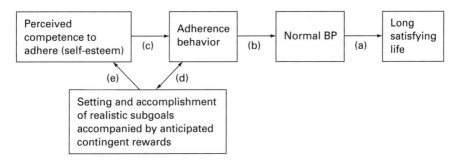

FIGURE 9–5   Model of major hypothesized predictors of adherence and their effects on blood pressure. Arrows between boxes indicate causal relationships. The letters on each arrow are used for reference in the text. *Source:* Caplan RD, Robinson EAR, French JRP, Caldwell JR, Shinn M: *Adhering to Medical Regimens: Pilot Experiments in Patient Education and Social Support.* Ann Arbor, MI: Institute for Social Research, Univ of Michigan, © 1976. Reprinted with permission.

note in the model presented by Caplan et al. is the bidirectional relationship between adherent behavior and goal setting and attainment *(D)*. Two subsequent expansions of this model were made by Caplan et al. (1976), but for brevity we have not included those here.

Several theorists in nursing have published the results of their theory synthesis work. Among these are the following theories: balance between analgesia and side effects in adults (Good & Moore, 1996); peaceful end of life (Ruland & Moore, 1998); acute pain management in infants and children (Huth & Moore, 1998); poststroke recovery (Easton, 1999); and synthesis of two theories related to nurses' communication patterns in the workplace (DeMarco, 2002). For example, Good and Moore (1996) drew their evidence base from practice guidelines on pain management for their theory synthesis. They used the strategy of statement synthesis to transform practice guidelines into statements suitable for theory synthesis. Three statements were synthesized from the guidelines. These were then organized in the resultant middle-range theory of balance of analgesia and side effects. They then stated assumptions and limits of the theory. The benefits of the integrated theory were a parsimonious presentation of diverse information related to the phenomena of pain management.

Finally, a synthesized theory proposed by Hall (1990) drew on participant observation, interviews, and clinical knowledge to formulate a theoretical model of recovery from alcoholism among lesbian women. She synthesized concepts about five tensions—that is, opposing qualities related dialectically in alcoholism recovery. These were (1) self: uniqueness/sameness, (2) affiliation: intimacy/intimidation, (3) power: authority/autonomy, (4) trajectory: determinism/determination, and (5) wholeness: integrity/disintegration. These concepts were incorporated into statements and a model of the recovery process in lesbian women. Power was postulated to be central; it interacts with self and affiliation tensions to influence the trajectory tension which then affects wholeness. Finally, the wholeness tension influences other tensions.

ADVANTAGES AND LIMITATIONS

The strength of theory synthesis as a strategy is the resultant integration of large amounts of discrete information about a topic. By using both linguistic and graphic modalities, synthesized theories can integrate and efficiently present multiple and complex relationships. Theory synthesis is a useful strategy for summarizing research findings relevant to educational, research, and practice spheres.

Theorists may need to increase their fluency with statistical concepts in order to make accurate discriminations about structural relationships between and among concepts in their evidence base. These discriminations include clarifying causal pathways among sets of variables.

Theory synthesis is built on the premise that theory development is an incremental and cumulative process. Although this may be true at certain levels of scientific development, this may not characterize those major advances in scientific thought that have occurred by making radical reorganizations of or departures from accumulated knowledge (Kuhn, 1962).

UTILIZING THE RESULTS OF THEORY SYNTHESIS

In the context of research, theory synthesis results lay bare the conceptual structure and linkages of extant knowledge about a phenomenon. This structural knowledge may then be used to ensure operational adequacy (Fawcett, 1999) of indicators and research procedures in empirically testing synthesized theory. Consequently, even a well-designed theoretical model needs to be empirically validated. Model or theory testing is needed to provide the sound empirical base desired of theories in a scientific discipline and profession. Testing may show that a model needs to be modified. If parts of a model repeatedly do not perform under rigorous tests (e.g., do not show expected relationships), then theorists have several alternatives. They may delete nonperforming variables, introduce new variables, or rethink the whole model. For example, if the model of transformational leadership were tested, it might need to be reworked. Perhaps gender-specific concepts (Eisler & Hersen, 2000) could be added to create separate models for men and women. As before, testing is needed to determine the merit of any changes in a model.

Development of synthesized theories may be useful in teaching complex content involving multiple concepts and their interrelationships. Often when such material is presented graphically as well as linguistically, it is easier both to teach and to learn. Students may also find it easier to retain complex relationships if they are given the opportunity to sketch out relationships embedded in text format.

Synthesized theories may help nurses in practice to examine the antecedents and consequences of a clinical phenomenon, or to plan patient services based on a coherent program theory. Designing preventive interventions may be facilitated by looking at the antecedents of a clinical problem. Tracing the way that each potential antecedent might be modified in an attempt to prevent undesired clinical problems, such as hospital readmissions after surgery, can suggest how present practice might be improved. This approach is also applicable to clinical problems outside the hospital context, as in home care and community agency settings.

SUMMARY

Because theory synthesis is based on empirical evidence, it enables a theorist to organize and integrate a wide variety of research information on a topic of interest. In theory synthesis, sets of concepts and discrete statements are organized into an interrelated system of statements with accompanying graphic representations. Theory synthesis may incorporate information from published research literature, direct statistical information, and qualitative research. Because theory synthesis may be used for several related purposes, deciding on the specific purpose depends on the balance among the theorist's interests, the use planned for the synthesized theory, and the amount and type of information available on a topic.

Three steps or phases are involved in theory synthesis: (1) specifying focal concepts for the synthesized theory, (2) reviewing the literature to identify factors related to the focal concepts and the relationships among these, and (3) organizing concepts and statements into an integrated and efficient representation of the phenomena of interest.

Theory synthesis allows a large amount of information to be efficiently organized. If quantitative data are involved, the use of the strategy requires some statistical sophistication of the part of the theorist. The strategy assumes an incremental approach to scientific progress.

PRACTICE EXERCISE

Obesity researchers, such as Hill and Peters (1998), have argued that modern life is at odds with our evolved human regulatory systems for taking in, storing, and expending energy. Specifically, factors such as the widespread availability of energy-dense foods and growing use of energy-sparing modern conveniences have led to the rapid onset of a national obesity epidemic in the United States (Mokdad, Bowman, Ford, et al., 2001; Mokdad, Serdula, Dietz, et al., 1999). One consequence of this has been growth in the number of people who are obese. Obesity, in turn, is predicted to lead to increased rates of many of its sequelae, such as cardiovascular disease, diabetes mellitus, gastric reflux syndrome, orthopedic problems, and certain cancers.

For this exercise, develop several statements regarding the antecedents and consequences of the obesity epidemic. Based on your statements, make a diagram synthesizing these statements into a model of the "epidemic of obesity."

When you have completed this exercise, compare your theoretical model with Figure 9–6. Although your model may not look exactly like ours, there should be some structural similarity to it.

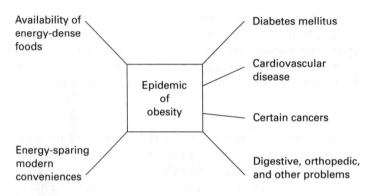

FIGURE 9–6   Model of the epidemic of obesity.

REFERENCES

Blalock HM. *Theory Construction: From Verbal to Mathematical Formulations.* Englewood Cliffs, NJ: Prentice Hall; 1969.

Caplan RD, Robinson EAR, French JRP, Caldwell JR, Shinn M. *Adhering to Medical Regimens: Pilot Experiments in Patient Education and Social Support.* Ann Arbor: Institute for Social Research, University of Michigan; 1976.

Causey R. Scientific progress. *Tex Eng Sci Mag.* 1969;6(1):22-29.

DeMarco R. Two theories/a sharper lens: the staff nurse voice in the workplace. *J Adv Nurs.* 2002;38:549-556.

Easton KL. The poststroke journey: from agonizing to owning. *Geriatr Nurs.* 1999;20:70-76.

Eisler RM, Hersen M, eds. *Handbook of Gender, Culture, and Health.* Mahwah, NJ: Erlbaum; 2000.

Fawcett J. *The Relationship of Theory and Research.* 3rd ed. Philadelphia, Penn: Davis; 1999.

Good M, Moore SM. Clinical practice guidelines as a new source of middle-range theory: focus on acute pain. *Nurs Outlook.* 1996;44:74-79.

Hall JM. Alcoholism recovery in lesbian women: a theory in development. *Scholar Inquiry Nurs Pract.* 1990;4:109-122.

Hempel CG. *Philosophy of Natural Science.* Englewood Cliffs, NJ: Prentice Hall; 1966.

Hill JO, Peters JC. Environmental contributions to the obesity epidemic. *Science.* 1998;280:1371-1374.

Huth MM, Moore SM. Prescriptive theory of acute pain management in infants and children. *J Soc Pediatr Nurses.* 1998;3:23-32.

Kuhn TS. *The Structure of Scientific Revolutions.* Chicago, Ill: University of Chicago Press; 1962.

Mokdad AH, Bowman BA, Ford ES, Vinicor F, Marks JS, Koplan JP. The continuing epidemics of obesity and diabetes in the United States. *JAMA.* 2001;286:1195-1200.

Mokdad AH, Serdula MK, Dietz WH, Bowman BA, Marks JS, Koplan JP. The spread of the obesity epidemic in the United States, 1991–1998. *JAMA.* 1999;282:1519-1522.

Ruland CM, Moore SM. Theory construction based on standards of care: a proposed theory of the peaceful end of life. *Nurs Outlook.* 1998;46:169-175.

Ward K. A vision for tomorrow: transformational nursing leaders. *Nurs Outlook.* 2002;50:121-126.

Zetterberg HL. *On Theory and Verification in Sociology.* Totowa, NJ: Bedminster Press; 1965.

ADDITIONAL READINGS
Readings in Theory Development

Blalock HM. *Theory Construction: From Verbal to Mathematical Formulations.* Englewood Cliffs, NJ: Prentice Hall; 1969.

Dubin R. *Theory Building.* New York, NY: Free Press; 1978.

Field M. Causal inferences in behavioral research. *Adv Nurs Sci.* 1979;2(1):81-93.

Hage J. *Techniques and Problems of Theory Construction in Sociology.* New York, NY: Wiley; 1972.

Lancaster W, Lancaster J. Models and model building in nursing. *Adv Nurs Sci.* 1981;3(3):31-42.

Mullins NC. *The Art of Theory: Construction and Use.* New York, NY: Harper & Row; 1971.

Reynolds PD. *A Primer in Theory Construction.* Indianapolis, Ind: Bobbs-Merrill; 1971.

Stember ML. Model building as a strategy for theory development. In: Chinn PL, ed. *Nursing Research Methodology.* Rockville, Md: Aspen; 1986.

Suppe F, Jacox AK. Philosophy of science and the development of nursing theory. In: Werley HH, Fitzpatrick JJ, eds. *Annual Review of Nursing Research.* Boston, Mass: Springer; 1985:241-267.

Zetterberg HL. *On Theory and Verification in Sociology.* Totowa, NJ: Bedminster Press; 1965.

Computer Software Adapted to Theory Building

arcs© is a program that "stores, tracks, and models relational data" (arcs© Product Information). It is available from Dr. Judith R. Graves, RN, PHD, FAAN, Adjunct Professor, Center for Research, Indiana University School of Nursing, Indianapolis, IN 46202; and President, Knowledge Research Group, Inc., 3230 Victory Circle, Gardnerville, NV 89410, USA; phone 775–266–4488; fax 775–266–0019; e-mail judithrgraves@hotmail.com.

10

Theory Derivation

Preliminary Note: Theory derivation is an easy strategy to learn if you are quick to see analogies. It is also an extremely efficient way to develop new theory. Nurses and other health care workers use analogy and metaphor frequently in their dealings with patients and clients. Analogy is often the basis for our health teaching. Thus, the derivation strategies are very popular with our students because the strategies are intuitive and easy for them to grasp. Some of the earliest work using derivation was done in the 1960s in education. We have drawn heavily on that work.

DEFINITION AND DESCRIPTION

Using analogy to obtain explanations or predictions about a phenomenon in one field from the explanations or predictions in another field is the basis for theory derivation (Maccia, Maccia, & Jewett, 1963). Thus, a theory (T_1) from one field of interest (F_1) offers some new insights to a theorist who then moves certain content or structural features into his or her own field of interest (F_2) to form a new theory (T_2). Theory derivation is an easy way to develop theory rapidly in a new field because all that is required is (1) the ability to see analogous dimensions of phenomena in two distinct fields of interest and (2) the ability to redefine and transpose the content and/or structure from Field 1 to Field 2 in a manner that adds significant insights about some phenomenon in Field 2 (Figure 10–1).

Seeing an analogy requires imagination and creativity; it is not a mechanical exercise. Theory derivation also requires the theorist to be able to redefine the concepts and statements so that they are meaningful in the new field. Because the two fields are obviously different, certain modifications will have to be made when transposing a theory from one to the other field. Two distinctions must be made here: the distinction between theory derivation and statement derivation, and the distinction between "borrowing" or sharing theory and theory derivation. Theory derivation is a process whereby a whole set of interrelated concepts or a whole structure is moved from one field to another and modified to fit the new field, whereas in statement derivation you move only *individual* isolated

148

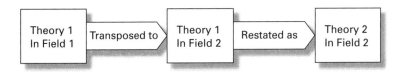

FIGURE 10–1   Process of theory derivation.

statements from one field to another and modify them. Statement derivation is on a smaller scale than theory derivation, although the actual steps in the process are similar.

When a theorist borrows or shares a theory, the theory is moved *unchanged* from one discipline to another. For example, we have used chemical, biological, and psychological theories in nursing for many years without any changes needing to be made in the original theories when they are applied in nursing. However, if we wished to *derive* a new theory to use in nursing from any of these fields, we would need to modify the concepts and/or the structure in those theories to fit our particular needs. Theories cannot be moved unchanged from one field to another as an example of theory derivation. True theory derivation requires that at least some modifications in content or structure be made.

PURPOSE AND USES

Theory derivation is particularly useful where no data are available or where new insights about a phenomenon are needed to inspire research and testing. Theory derivation is also useful when a theorist has a set of concepts that are somehow related to each other, but has no structural way to represent those relationships. (See Chapter 7 for more detailed description of structure derivation.) In this case, the theorist might find that some other field of interest has a structure in one of its theories that is analogous to the relationships of the concepts in which he or she is interested. The theorist may use the derivation strategy appropriately by adopting and adapting the structure to fit the concepts being considered. This adds to the body of knowledge in the theorist's field in a significant and rapid way that might not have happened for some time without the derivation strategy. An example of this is Nierenberg's classic use of Maslow's hierarchical structure of needs to derive a theory of negotiation (1968, 1973).

When a theorist has some ideas about the basic structure of a phenomenon but has no concepts to describe it, theory derivation is also very useful. Another theory in a different field may provide the theorist with a set of analogous concepts that can help describe the phenomenon, if modified slightly. Again, this procedure rapidly adds to the body of knowledge in the theorist's own field. We used one example of this strategy in Chapter 4, where Roy and Roberts (1981) developed the concepts of focal, contextual, and residual stimuli in patient assessment from a psychophysics theory by Helson.

Several examples of theory derivation come quickly to mind when we consider systems theory. Many of our nursing models in their original form have been direct derivations from systems theory—Roy and Roberts (1981); Neuman (1980); Erickson, Tomlin, and Swain (1983); and others have significant aspects of theory derivation systems in them.

PROCEDURES FOR THEORY DERIVATION

Although the actual process may not occur sequentially, theory derivation can be discussed as a series of sequential steps. However, theory derivation is really more an iterative process. That is, the theorist goes back and forth between some or all of the steps until the level of sophistication of the theory is acceptable.

There are several basic steps in theory derivation:

1. Be cognizant of the level of theory development in your own field of interest and evaluate the scientific usefulness of any such development. This implies that you are or will arrange to be thoroughly familiar with the literature on the topic of interest. If your evaluation leads you to believe that none of the current theories are suitable or useful, then theory derivation can proceed.

2. Read widely in nursing and in other fields for ideas while allowing imagination and creativity free reign. Reading widely enables you to understand ways of putting theory together and gives you insight into new concepts and structures you may not have thought about before. Allowing your imagination and creativity free reign opens your mind to possible analogies. Discovering analogies is often done accidentally or as a creative intuitive leap rather than systematically.

3. Select a parent theory to use for derivation. The parent theory should be chosen because it offers a new and insightful way of explaining or predicting about a phenomenon in the theorist's field of interest. The parent theory may be, and often is, from another field or discipline, but a nursing theory may also be used. Any theory that provides you with a useful analogy can be chosen. However, just any theory won't do. Many theories will shed no light at all on the concepts of interest or fail to provide useful structure for the concepts and are therefore worthless to the theorist. Keep in mind here that the whole parent theory may not be needed to form the new theory. Only those portions that are analogous and therefore relevant need be used.

4. Identify what content and/or structure from the parent theory is to be used. Perhaps only the concepts or only the statements are analogous, but not the overall structure. Or perhaps the structure is perfect but the parent concepts and statements are not. Perhaps the theorist needs concepts and statements as well as structure. In the derivation strategy, the theorist is free to choose what best fits the needs of the situation.

5. Develop or redefine any new concepts or statements from the content or structure of the parent theory in terms of the phenomenon of interest to

the theorist. This is the hardest part of theory derivation, but also the most fun. It requires creativity and thoughtfulness on the part of the theorist. Basically, the concepts or structure that is borrowed from the parent field is modified in such a way that it becomes meaningful in the theorist's field. Often the modifications are small, but occasionally they will need to be substantial before the theory makes sense in the new setting.

Illustrations are often clearer than verbal explanations, so we are providing several brief examples of theory derivation. Let us begin with a classic example. Maccia, Maccia, and Jewett (1963) used both concepts and structure of a theory of eye blinks to derive a theory of education. Because they were some of the first scholars to explicitly use derivation for theory development, we have included an example from their work. Listed below are a few of the principles and their derivations from Maccia, Maccia, and Jewett.

Parent Theory Statements	Maccia and Colleagues' Derivation
1. Either the eyes are or are not covered by lids.	1. The student is either distracted or attentive.
2. Blinking functions to protect the eyes from contact and to rest the retina and the ocular muscles.	2. Distraction functions to protect the student from mental stress and to rest from mental effort.
3. Blinking may be either reflexive or nonreflexive	3. Distraction may be either voluntary or involuntary.
4. Reflex blinking may be inhibited by a fixation object or by drugs.	4. Involuntary distraction may be inhibited by attention cues or by drugs.
5. Nonreflexive blinking may occur if seeing is unwanted.	5. Voluntary distraction may occur if learning is unwanted.

In an early nursing example of derivation, Wewers and Lenz (1987) derived a theory of relapse among ex-smokers from Cronkite and Moos's (1980) theory of posttreatment functioning of alcoholics. Wewers and Lenz primarily used content derivation, but also derived a simplified structure. Listed below are three propositions from Cronkite and Moos with the derivations made by Wewers and Lenz. In some cases we have adapted the wording of the propositions to show the derivations more clearly.

Because there was already a large amount of literature available on smoking, Wewers and Lenz adopted propositions in their derivation that fit knowledge specifically about smoking. This is an excellent example of how to use the strategy flexibly in theory-building efforts.

Parent Theory Statements	Wewers and Lenz's (1987) Derivations
1. Pretreatment symptoms such as alcohol consumption, type of drinker, depression, and occupational functioning are related to alcohol treatment outcomes (p. 48).	1. Pretreatment symptoms such as cigarette consumption and type of smoker are related to smoking relapse (p. 48).
2. "Stressful life events were negatively associated with some aspects of recovery" (p. 49).	2. "Both the social contextual stressor of major life events and the internal stressor of craving" are associated with smoking relapse (p. 49).
3. Family environment is "weakly related to alcohol recovery" (p. 49).	3. "Long term smoking cessation is associated with having family members who are nonsmokers or who had previously been able to quit smoking" (p. 49).

Mishel's (1990) reconceptualization of the uncertainty of illness theory provides another nursing example. Mishel used the content and structure of chaos theory to help her describe the outcome portion of her model more clearly. We have selected three statements to illustrate how the derivation was made. In an effort to be as clear and succinct as possible, we have at times restated the propositions to make the analogies more obvious.

Parent Theory Statements	Mishel's Derivation
1. "In a far-from equilibrium [sic] system, the sensitivity of the initial condition is such that small changes yield huge effects and the system reorganizes itself in multiple ways" (p. 259).	1. "Abiding uncertainty can dismantle the existing cognitive structures that give meaning to everyday events. This loss of meaning throws the person into a state of confusion and disorganization" (p. 260).
2. "Fluctuations in the system can become so powerful . . . that they shatter the preexisting organization" (p. 259).	2. "If the uncertainty factors of disease or illness multiply rapidly past a critical value, the stability of the personal system can no longer be taken for granted" (p. 260).
3. "Auto-catalytic processes result in a product whose presence encourages further production of itself. . . producing disorder" (p. 259).	3. "The existence of uncertainty in one area of illness often feeds back on itself and generates further uncertainty in other illness-related events" (p. 260).

Theory derivation can happen using two widely disparate fields. Or insight can come from a closely related field. It is the theorist's creativity and intuition that provide the insight into the analogy.

A theorist does not have to derive both concepts and structure. Derivation can be used only for concepts or only for structure. Let us examine one example in which only concepts were used and another example in which only structure was used. Jones (2001) used only concepts to derive a theory about nursing time based on Adam's (1995) alternatives to clock/calendar time. Below are Adam's parent theory concepts with definitions and Jones's derivation. For other examples see the references under Additional Readings at the end of this chapter.

Parent Theory Statements	Jones's Derivation on Nursing Time
1. Temporality—"the cycle of life and death that occurs against the backdrop of unidirectional time" (p. 155).	1. Temporality—"There are unlimited amounts of parallel and cyclical time frames within which nurses exist simultaneously and within each frame we organize, plan, and regulate our lives" (p. 154).
2. Timing—is "when" time but clock and calendar times are not the only points of reference in determining "when" for scheduling, synchronization, allocation of resources, etc.	2. Timing—"Timing in . . . nursing is dependent on multiple considerations, based on past, present, and future times" (p. 156).
3. Tempo—Time may seem to advance at varying speeds, for example, "when we speak of time moving quickly or slowly" (p. 156).	3. Tempo—"Processes in the health services are mutually implicated in how much is achieved within a given timeframe in the timing of actions and in the temporality of existence" (p. 156).

Teel, Meek, McNamara, and Watson (1997), on the other hand, first synthesized four different theories and then used the four theories' structures to derive a new theory of symptom interpretation. Below we have attempted to denote the various parent theory statements beside the derivations that Teel et al. made from them.

Parent Theories Statements	Teel and Colleagues' Derivation
	(*Note:* Teel et al. sometimes formed a new proposition from more than one statement in the parent field. We have tried to indicate this by positioning the derived statements between the two parent statements.)
Barsalou (1989) Theory of Knowledge Structure	
1. "Knowledge structures are basic units of human information that undergird memory and intelligence" (p. 177). "Forms of knowledge structures are definitions, exemplars, prototypes, and mental models" (p. 177).	1. "Definitions, exemplars, prototypes, and mental models are associated with symptom recognition and assessment" (p. 177).
Leventhal, Myer, & Nerenz (1980) Common Sense Representation of Illness Model	
2. "Symptoms are integral to overall illness representation" (p. 176).	2. "An individual's knowledge of a symptom and the meaning attached to it are critical to understanding outcomes relative to the symptom" (p. 176).
3. "Symptoms are key elements in illness diagnosis" (p. 176).	3. "Disturbance awareness is recognizing that something is different from the normal pattern or becoming alert to a change in how one feels" (p. 176).
Tversky & Kahneman (1982, 1983) Propositions About Reasoning	
4. "Human judgments are known to diverge from rules of logic and probability, particularly in the presence of uncertainty" (p. 178). "Use of judgment heuristics is the dominant mode of human reasoning" (p. 178).	4. "Familiarity with a symptom prompts an individual to preferentially categorize symptoms that are like the typical symptom pattern" (p. 178).

Lang (1977, 1985) Psychophysiology of Fear and Anxiety	
5. "Knowledge structures are activated when a critical number of stored stimulus informational elements are matched by incoming stimuli" (p. 177).	5. "One's knowledge structures support a tendency to respond in specific ways to specific stimulus patterns" (p. 178).

Remember, derived theories are constructed in the context of discovery. The theories thus developed have no validity until they are subjected to empirical testing in the context of justification. Even if the theory is extremely relevant to practice or research, it must first be validated before it can be used. Several methods that may be used to test theories are presented in Chapter 12. Additional help may be found in the research references included here and in several other chapters.

ADVANTAGES AND LIMITATIONS

Theory derivation is a reasonably easy and quick way to obtain theory in new areas of interest. It is an exciting exercise in that it requires the theorist to use creativity and imagination in seeing analogies from one field and modifying them for use in a new field. In addition, theory derivation provides a way of arriving at explanation and prediction about a phenomenon where there may be little or no information, literature, or formal studies available.

One disadvantage is that the theorist must be familiar with a number of fields of interest other than his or her own. This implies reading widely and being constantly on the alert for new and profitable analogies. In addition, the theorist must be thoroughly familiar with the literature and current thinking about his or her particular area of interest. Otherwise, when the time comes to draw an analogy, the theorist will have difficulty choosing appropriate boundaries for the new theory.

Finally, novice theorists often become so excited about their new generalizations that they fail to take into account any dissimilarities, or dis-analogies, present in the parent theory. These dis-analogies should at least be considered for any valuable information that they might provide in the "new" theory. The dis-analogies may give further insight into the phenomenon or may provide useful "red flags" of trouble ahead.

UTILIZING THE RESULTS OF THEORY DERIVATION

The uses of theory derivation are to provide structure when only concepts are available, to provide concepts when only structure is available, or to provide both concepts and structure as an efficient way to begin theory development. The results of theory derivation are easily used in nursing education, practice, research, and theory development.

Theory derivation is an excellent way to obtain a theoretical framework for curriculum building in education. In addition, it can be used as a teaching tool with graduate students as a way to introduce them to theorizing in general. It is relatively easy to learn and fun to do as a group exercise. (To make the idea of "theory building" less scary for young students we often ask them first to derive a new theory that has to do with their daily lives rather than nursing. When they are successful at this, we then ask them to derive a nursing theory.)

Theory derivation can provide significant new insights for clinical practice. Clinicians can provide themselves with a useful theoretical framework to guide their practice by using the results of theory derivation.

Theory derivation is also a simple way to design a conceptual model for a research program. Moving concepts and/or structure from the parent field with appropriate changes yields a rich source of potential hypotheses for study, as Wewers and Lenz demonstrated. It is a very efficient strategy for achieving a body of knowledge about a phenomenon.

SUMMARY

Theory derivation is an excellent way of obtaining rapid theory development in a new field because it uses analogy to obtain explanations or predictions about a phenomenon in one field from explanations or predictions in another field. Both concepts and structure can be moved from the parent field to the new one, undergoing modifications along the way.

There are five steps to theory derivation: (1) become thoroughly familiar with the topic of interest; (2) read widely in other fields, allowing your imagination to help you find useful analogies; (3) select a parent theory to use for derivation; (4) identify what content and/or structure from the parent theory is to be used; and (5) modify or redefine new concepts and/or statements in terms of the phenomenon of interest. Once the new theory has been formulated, it must be tested empirically to validate that the new concepts and structure actually reflect reality in the new field.

Theory derivation is an easy and fast means of constructing new theories. One disadvantage is that the theorist must be widely read in several fields as well as his or her own field. In addition, the theorist must remember to consider the dissimilarities as well as the similarities between the parent field and the new field.

At this point in our development of a knowledge base, theory derivation is a highly workable strategy for nursing. It provides a means of rapid acquisition of theory with meaningful content. If carefully done and carefully tested, derived theories could play an immediate role in the development of scientific knowledge in nursing.

PRACTICE EXERCISES

Below is a list of 17 relational statements from a general systems theory for behavioral science (Miller, 1955). Using the derivation strategy in this chapter, construct a new theory for nursing in your own particular area of clinical interest. You don't have to include all 17 statements. Choose the ones most relevant to your area of interest. Remember that an open system is one that is bounded in space and time and that exchanges energy and information with its subsystems and with its environment (suprasystem).

a. Greater energy is required for transmission across a boundary than for transmission within the environment or within a subsystem.
b. Spread of energy or information throughout systems is quantitatively comparable.
c. There is a constant systematic distortion—or alteration—between inputs of energy or information into the system and outputs from the system.
d. The distortion of a system is the sum of the effects of processes that subtract from the input to reduce the strains in subsystems or add to the output to reduce the strains.
e. When variables in a system return to equilibrium after stress, the rate of return and the strength of the restorative forces are stronger than a linear function of the amount of displacement from the equilibrium point.
f. Living systems respond to continuously increasing stress first by a lag in response, then by overcompensation, then by collapse of the system.
g. Systems that survive employ the least expensive defenses against stress first and increasingly more expensive ones later.
h. Systems that survive perform at an optimum efficiency for maximum power output, which is always less than maximum efficiency.
i. When a system's negative feedback discontinues, its steady state vanishes, its boundaries disappear, and the system ends.
j. The output of a system is always less than its input.
k. Decentralization of the maintenance of variables in equilibrium is always more expensive of energy than centralization, although it may increase utility.
l. As decentralization increases, subsystems increasingly act without the benefit of information available elsewhere in the system.
m. The more subsystems there are in efficient systems, the more variables they can maintain in equilibrium.
n. The more subsystems there are in efficient systems, the more subsystems whose destruction will cause the system to collapse.
o. When reduction of several strains is not possible simultaneously, the order in which they are reduced in systems that survive is from strongest to weakest, if the effort required for reduction is the same.
p. Up to a maximum, the more energy in a system devoted to information processing, the more likely the system is to survive.
q. When one living species feeds on another in a given suprasystem, and both species continue to survive, an oscillation of numbers of predators and prey occurs around an equilibrium point.

Just for fun, we derived a theory about graduate students in nursing. You may wish to compare your theory with ours below. We chose to use only a few statements to give you an example of how derivation might work. We have used the same alphabetical notation as the parent theory statements to help you identify where our statements come from.

a. Graduate students in nursing communicate with each other more efficiently than with their professors.

c. When graduate students are told the course requirements at the beginning of a course, they will ask for clarification of those requirements before midterm.

f. 1. The nearer exams or deadlines approach, the more study groups are formed.

    2. As exams or deadlines approach, the illness rate in students increases.

o. When several projects are due at once, graduate students will complete the most difficult project first.

p. The more reading and thinking done by the student, the more likely he or she is to complete the degree.

j. Graduate students must complete a full curriculum in order to have enough skills to complete a thesis or dissertation.

i. When the final thesis or dissertation defense is completed, the student graduates.

REFERENCES

Adam B. *Timewatch: The Social Analysis of Time.* Cambridge, England: Polity Press; 1995.

Barsalou LW. Intraconcept similarity and its implications for interconcept similarity. In: Vosniadou S, Ortony A, eds. *Similarity and Analogical Reasoning.* New York, NY: Cambridge University Press; 1989:76-121.

Cronkite RC, Moos RH. Determinants of the post-treatment functioning of alcoholic patients: a conceptual framework. *J Consult Clin Psychol.* 1980;48:305-316.

Erickson HC, Tomlin EM, Swain MAP. *Modeling and Role Modeling: A Theory and Paradigm of Nursing.* Englewood Cliffs, NJ: Prentice Hall; 1983.

Jones AR. Time to think: temporal considerations in nursing practice and research. *J Adv Nurs.* 2001;33(2):150-158.

Lang PJ. Imagery in therapy: an information processing analysis of fear. *Behav Ther.* 1977;8(5):862-886.

Lang PJ. The cognitive psychophysiology of emotion: fear and anxiety. In: Tuma AH, Maser J, eds. *Anxiety and the Anxiety Disorders.* Hillsdale, NJ: Erlbaum; 1985:7-30.

Leventhal H, Meyer D, Nerenz D. The common sense representation of illness danger. In: Rachman S, ed. *Contributions to Medical Psychology and Health.* New York, NY: Pergamon Press: 1980.

Maccia ES, Maccia GS, Jewett RE. *Construction of Educational Theory Models.* Cooperative Research Project #1632. Columbus: Ohio State University Research Foundation; 1963.

Miller JG. Toward a general theory for behavioral science. *Am Psychol.* 1955;10(9):513-531.

Mishel MH. Reconceptualization of the uncertainty of illness theory. *Image.* 1990;22(4): 256-262.

Neuman B. The Betty Neuman health care systems model: a total person approach to patient problems. In: Riehl JP, Roy C, eds. *Conceptual Models for Nursing Practice*. 2nd ed. New York, NY: Appleton-Century-Crofts; 1980.

Nierenberg GI. *Fundamentals of Negotiating*. New York, NY: Hawthorne; 1973.

Nierenberg GI. *The Art of Negotiating*. New York, NY: Hawthorne; 1968.

Roy C, Roberts SL. *Theory Construction in Nursing: An Adaptation Model*. Englewood Cliffs, NJ: Prentice Hall; 1981.

Teel CS, Meek P, McNamara AM, Watson L. Perspectives unifying symptom interpretation. *Image*. 1997;29(2):175-181.

Tversky A, Kahneman D. Extensional versus intuitive reasoning: the conjunction fallacy in probability judgment. *Psychol Rev.* 1983;90(4):293-315.

Tversky A, Kahneman D. Judgments of and by representativeness. In: Kahneman D, Slovic P, Tversky A, eds. *Judgement under Uncertainty: Heuristics and Biases*. New York, NY: Cambridge University Press; 1982:89-90.

Wewers ME, Lenz E. Relapse among ex-smokers: an example of theory derivation. *Adv Nurs Sci.* 1987;9(2):44-53.

ADDITIONAL READINGS

Burr JW. *Theory Construction and the Sociology of the Family*. New York, NY: Wiley; 1973.

Challey PS. Theory derivation in moral development. *Nurs Health Care*. 1990;11(6):302-306.

Comley AL, Beard MT. Toward a derived theory of patient satisfaction. *J Theory Construct Test*. 1998;2(2):44-50.

Condon EH. Theory derivation: application to nursing . . . the caring perspective within professional nurse role development. *J Nurs Educ*. 1986; 25(4):156-159.

Henderson JS, Hamilton P, Vicenza AE. Chaos theory in nursing publications: retrospective and prospective views. *Complexity Chaos Nurs*. 1995;2(1):36-40.

Kaplan A. *The Conduct of Inquiry*. New York, NY: Chandler; 1964.

Leventhal H. Symptom reporting: a focus on process. In: McHugh S, Vallias TM, eds. *Illness Behavior: A Multidisciplinary Model*. New York, NY: Plenum Press; 1986.

Leventhal H, Nerenz DR, Strauss A. Self-regulation and the mechanisms for symptom appraisal. In: Mechanic D, ed. *Symptoms, Illness Behavior and Help-seeking*. New York, NY: Prodist; 1982:55-86.

Miller JG. *Living Systems*. New York, NY: McGraw-Hill; 1978.

Olson RW. *The Art of Creative Thinking: A Practical Guide*. New York, NY: Barnes Noble; 1980.

11

Theory Analysis

Preliminary Note: *We have been delightedly surprised at how many theories are undergoing analysis and revision over the last several years. This is a very encouraging trend. It reveals the rapid nature of the development of the science of nursing. There are also many more middle-range theories under development. They provide the discipline with a rich source of potential knowledge about how nursing "works" and how effective and efficient nursing care is. We encourage researchers, advanced practice nurses, staff nurses, and students to examine any theory they intend to teach or to use in practice to be sure it is a valid theory and is reliable in its description, explanation, prediction, and prescription or control.*

DEFINITION AND DESCRIPTION

Theory is usually constructed to express a unique, unifying idea about a phenomenon that answers previously unanswered questions and provides new insights into the nature of the phenomenon. A theory attempts to establish a parsimonious, precise example, or model, of the real world or the world as it is experienced. Thus, theory is defined as a set of interrelated relational statements about a phenomenon that is useful for description, explanation, prediction, and prescription or control (Chinn & Jacobs, 1987; Dickoff, James, & Wiedenbach, 1968a, 1968b; Hardy, 1974; Hempel, 1965; Reynolds, 1971).

A theory purporting to describe, explain, or predict something should provide the reader with a clear idea of what the phenomenon is and does, what events affect it, and how it affects other phenomena. Therefore, theory analysis is the systematic examination of the theory for meaning, logical adequacy, usefulness, generality, parsimony, and testability.

In theory analysis, as in all analysis strategies, the theory is broken down into parts. Each is examined individually as it relates to every other. In addition, the theoretical structure as a whole is examined to determine such things as validity and approximation to the real world.

PURPOSE AND USES

Theory analysis allows you to examine both the strengths and the weaknesses of a theory. In addition, a theory analysis may determine the need for additional development or refinement of the original theory.

Theory analysis provides a systematic, objective way of examining a theory that may lead to insights and formulations previously undiscovered. This then adds to the body of knowledge in the nursing discipline. As Popper pointed out in a classic work (1965), science is interested in novel ideas and interesting theories because their very novelty or interest prompts the scientist to put them to empirical test. Theory analysis offers one way of determining "what" needs to be put to the test and often suggests "how" it can be done.

A formal theory analysis is relevant only if the theory has the possibility of being useful in either an educational, clinical practice, or research setting. If the theory demonstrates no potential for usefulness, then the analysis becomes a futile exercise. It has been our experience that the primary purpose for conducting a theory analysis prior to using that theory in education or clinical practice is to discover the strong points the theory offers to guide practice. However, a theory analysis for the purposes of research usually focuses on the weak points or the unsubstantiated linkages among its concepts. The reason for this distinction is that the analysis provides evidence the researcher needs to justify conducting a study concerning new or unclear relationships within the original theory.

Understanding is the main aim of **analysis**. To truly understand something we must put aside our own values and biases and look objectively at the object of analysis. Because a theory analysis is both systematic and objective, it provides a way to examine the content and structure of a theory without being influenced by subjective evaluation. Leaving our personal values out of the analysis allows us to see the theory more clearly, and the original theorist's values will become more evident.

The main aim of **evaluation**, on the other hand, is decision and/or action. Here, our own values and biases become important to the outcome. Evaluation of theory should only be done *after* a thorough analysis is made. Then, we should feel free to evaluate the theory's potential contribution to scientific knowledge and to make judgments about its worth in establishing a basis for making decisions or taking action (Fawcett, 1980, 1989, 1993, 1995, 2000).

PROCEDURES FOR THEORY ANALYSIS

The steps in theory analysis were synthesized from the works of Popper (1961, 1965), Reynolds (1971), Hardy (1974), Fawcett (1980, 1989, 2000), and Chinn and Jacobs (1987). Despite their age, these authors' works collectively formed the existing foundation of knowledge in theory development. Without their pioneering efforts, nursing theory development would be seriously behind and this book might not exist.

There are six steps in theory analysis: (1) identify the origins of the theory, (2) examine the meaning of the theory, (3) analyze the logical adequacy of the theory, (4) determine the usefulness of the theory, (5) define the degree of generalizability and the parsimony of the theory, and (6) determine the testability of the theory. Each of these steps will first be defined briefly and then discussed in detail.

The **origins** of a theory refer to its initial development. The analyst investigates what prompted its development, whether the theory is inductive or deductive in form, and if evidence exists to support or refute the theory.

The **meaning** (Hardy, 1974) of a theory has to do with the theory's concepts and how they relate to each other. Essentially, the meaning is reflected in the language of the theory and calls for a careful examination of the specific language used by the original theorist.

The **logical adequacy** (Hardy, 1974) of a theory denotes the logical structure of the concepts and statements independent of their meaning. The analyst looks for any logical fallacies in the structure of the theory and examines the accuracy with which predictions can be made from the theory.

The **usefulness** of a theory concerns how practical and helpful the theory is to the discipline in providing a sense of understanding or predictable outcomes. A theory that provides a practitioner with realistic guides to practice so that Intervention A consistently leads to Patient Behavior B, for instance, is obviously more useful than one that does not.

Generalizability, or **transferability**, explains the extent to which generalizations can be made from the theory. The more widely the theory can be applied, the more generalizable it becomes.

Parsimony refers to how simply and briefly a theory can be stated while still being complete in its explanation of the phenomenon in question. Many mathematical theories are parsimonious, for example, because they offer an explanation in only a few equations. Social science theories are rarely parsimonious, on the other hand, because they deal with such complex human phenomena that they defy mathematical expression.

Testability has to do with whether the theory can be supported by empirical data. If a theory cannot generate hypotheses that can be subjected to empirical research, it is not testable.

We believe that all of these six steps are important to a complete theory analysis. Some authors disagree. Fawcett (2000) states that the last two steps—determining parsimony and testability—are really related to theory evaluation. Granted, when one completes the analysis and begins to evaluate the theory, one may place heavier values on some of the steps than on others. But, if a theory has poorly defined and inconsistently used concepts, for instance, it will not be capable of test, will not have parsimony, and will not be useful. The value assigned to a theory rests primarily on what the analysis reveals, but it also reflects one's own feelings and biases to a certain extent. This is to be expected; no scientist can ever be completely objective. We will now more thoroughly discuss each of the analysis steps.

Origins

The first step is to determine what prompted the development of the theory. Sometimes the theorist will offer an explicit explanation. Otherwise, the analyst may only be able to surmise this from the context of the discussion. Understanding the origin of a theory and the purpose for which it was developed often prove very helpful to the analyst in understanding how the theory was put together and why. Begin by reading the theory carefully, identifying the major ideas or concepts, and isolating the relational statements. In addition, find out if the theory was developed deductively (from a more general law) or inductively (from data). If the theory was developed from another theory or from some other hypothesis, it can be considered deductive in origin. It can be considered inductive in origin if observations of relationships from data, literature, or clinical practice generated the theory. Later when determining its logical adequacy, the inductive or deductive form of origin will be important. Finally, it is often helpful to identify any underlying assumptions on which the theory is built. These underlying assumptions can be important to interpretation and when considering the usefulness of the theory.

Meaning

Examining meaning and logical adequacy are the lengthy processes in a theory analysis, but also the most valuable. Meaning, in theory analysis, refers to the semantics of the theory. An analyst must examine the language used in the theory by looking at the concepts and statements within it. The steps are: identify the concepts, examine their definitions and use, identify the statements, and examine the relationships among concepts as demonstrated in the statements.

Identify Concepts   Look for the major ideas in the theory. All relevant terms that reflect those ideas should be clearly stated and defined. It is often difficult to identify the major concepts in an elaborate verbal model. Probably the best approach is to read with a pencil and paper at hand. As new terms appear, write them down with their definitions, if given. This saves time in the long run and makes it very clear where definitions are missing.

Determine whether each concept is primitive, concrete, or abstract. As described in Chapters 2 and 5, primitive terms are those names for concepts that derive their meanings from common experience in the discipline and can only be defined by using examples (Wilson, 1969). Concrete concepts must be directly measurable and are restricted by time and space. Abstract concepts are not limited by time or space and may not be directly measurable. Classifying the concepts in this way will aid the analyst in assessing the concrete or abstract nature of the entire theory.

Examine Definitions and Use   There are four possible options in regard to definitions: a theoretical definition, an operational definition, a descriptive definition, and no definition.

A **theoretical** definition uses other theoretical terms to define a concept and place it within the context of the theory but does not specify any operational rules for classifying or measuring it. A theoretical definition is usually fairly abstract and may use lower-order concepts to define higher-order ones. The most important criterion, though, is the lack of measurement specification in the definition.

A theoretical definition may provide the theorist with a way of expressing the richness of the concept within the theory and the means for classifying a phenomenon as either an example of the concept or not, but an **operational** definition provides the means for measuring the concept in question.

Operational definitions are useful in research but often artificially limit the concept. It is useful to the analyst, however, if both types of definitions are formulated for the major theoretical concepts. It is also very important to be sure that the operational definitions accurately reflect the theoretical definitions.

A **descriptive** definition, one that simply lists or describes the attributes of a concept much as in a dictionary, says nothing about the context in which the concept is used, nor does it specify operational measures. Having a descriptive definition is better than the last option, **no definitions** at all, but provides very limited data to the analyst. When only limited definitions are available, the analyst may find it difficult to make a truly objective analysis and equally difficult to use the theory for the purpose intended. When a theory contains only descriptive definitions or no definitions, it is often in a *very* early stage of development. It will be valuable if the analyst can make thoughtful suggestions about how further development should proceed.

The major concern in considering the way in which the concepts are used, is with consistency of use; that is, whether or not the theorist uses the concepts consistently, *as they are defined,* throughout the theory. This is vital information for anyone who proposes to apply the theory. If a theorist defines a concept in one way and then subtly, or not so subtly, alters the meaning as the theory develops, then all the formulations using that concept become suspect until the ambiguity of the definition can be cleared up. Otherwise, the analyst may attempt to predict outcomes from an early statement in a theory only to find that a later statement contradicts those same outcomes.

Additional research work regarding a theory may cause changes to be made in concept definitions or even in whole sections of a theory. It is to be expected that some refinements should be made. However, when such changes are necessitated, then the initial studies using the original concepts may not be useful in the support of the theory. They may need to be repeated and the initial relational statements retested for validity using the new concept definitions.

Identify Statements   Once the major concepts and definitions in the theory have been identified and examined, the analyst then concentrates specifically on relational statements. Relational statements identify the ways the concepts relate to each other. This process is not always easy, especially in elaborate verbal theories. Refer to the major concepts identified in the previous step when postulating relationships among them.

Look for explicit relational statements first. If you are dealing with research reports, you may look in the results section for the major relational statements. At other times, it may be necessary to start with the hypothesis section and work forward to the data analysis in order to find the relationships. Then go back and look for any relationships that may be implied or alluded to by the author or demonstrated but not reported in the tables or data analysis section.

When working from a verbal explanation written in non-research-report format, such as a descriptive article or a book chapter, it is often best to identify each concept as it appears along with any concepts that lie close to it on the page. Read carefully to see if association between any of the concepts is mentioned. Often the last few paragraphs or the summary of the article or chapter will offer some relationships, although we have found that summaries often give only the major relationships. Therefore, using summaries alone often leaves much of the richness of the theory in obscurity and hinders the analysis. For an excellent example of identifying statements and examining their relationships, see Cooley's (1999) analysis of the trajectory theory of chronic illness management.

Examine Relationships   Determining what types of relationships are specified, what boundaries are present, and whether the statements are used consistently is the first task in examining the relationships among concepts as demonstrated in the statements. In addition, the analyst must assess whether or not each statement has any valid empirical support. For the purpose of theory analysis, determining types of relationships will refer to questions of causation, association, and linearity. (For a more detailed method of statement analysis, refer to Chapter 8.)

As discussed in Chapter 8, *causal* relationships are those that specify that one concept always occurs as a direct result of the other concept. If any probability exists in the relationship whatsoever, it is not a true causal relationship (Hardy, 1974).

Associational relationships are those that specify that two concepts are related positively, negatively, or in no known way. This means that there is correlation between the two concepts but not causation. A positive association (+) indicates that both concepts vary together; that is, if one increases so does the other. A negative association (−) indicates that the concepts vary inversely; that is, as one concept increases, the other concept decreases. When two concepts occur simultaneously but there is no known relationship, the statement is given a question mark (?) as designation.

Linearity is assumed until proven otherwise. It is by far the easiest relationship to determine and test. Linearity assumes that a change in one variable or concept quickly produces an arithmetic change in the other concept or variable. When the correlation coefficients are calculated, the correlation will be strong and the slope of best fit a straight line.

There are other types of relational linkages, however, that can be determined either by deduction or by using data analysis, such as curvilinearity or power curves (Hage, 1972). The most difficult one to determine by analysis is the curvilinear linkage. Curvilinearity assumes that as one concept increases, the other concept also increases until a certain point is reached; then the second concept begins to decrease. The classic example of curvilinearity is the inverted U-shaped curve discussed in Chapter 7. Curvilinearity may be deduced by examining the formal theoretical and relational statements, or it may be determined by statistical analysis of data. If there are small but significant correlation coefficients among the data it is often useful to subject them to nonlinear analysis strategies to determine if the relationships are nonlinear.

The power curve shows an incremental relationship among concepts. That is, if one concept is shown to increase or decrease by a certain amount, the second concept changes at an accelerated rate in either a positive or a negative direction. Power curves are often called exponential curves because the changes in the second concept are often expressed mathematically in terms of exponents. Many of the system theories that use "inputs" and "outputs" also use power curves, as do some of the developmental and learning theories. Most power curves represent extensive periods (20 years or more) because they must take into account minor fluctuations and individual differences.

Next, determine what boundaries are present for the theory. Boundaries have to do with the actual content of the theory. Some theories have a very narrow focus and their boundaries, or limits, are clearly determined. In effect, a theory with narrow boundaries states exactly how far it can go in explaining specific phenomena and clarifying where the theory starts and stops. For example, a theory would have narrow boundaries if it addressed only a specific type of preoperative teaching for adults facing abdominal surgery in an American hospital.

A middle-range theory will have somewhat wider boundaries and will be more abstract than a narrow theory. The content may be very specific, but its application will encompass a wider group of events than the narrow theory. An example might be a theory that speaks to several predictable effects from two preoperative teaching strategies on adult surgical patients.

A theory with wide boundaries is highly abstract, covers a large content area, and is applicable in a large number of cases. To extend our preoperative teaching example a bit further, a theory with wide boundaries might reflect the effects of any preoperative teaching strategies on any preoperative patients from any cultural background, regardless of age or diagnosis.

Next, determine if the statements are used consistently. Look at all the statements: relational as well as existence and definitional. The theorist should use the statements in exactly the same way at all times. If this is not done, the theory loses credibility and becomes invalid for systematic use.

Finally, assess the empirical support for the statements. Is there any? If not, the theory will have less validity than one that does. If research or empirical evidence exists to support the statements, the analyst must evaluate the strength of the evidence. If the research studies are too numerous to review thoroughly, a generous sampling is permissible.

Determine from the reading how much research supports or refutes the statements in the theory. To do this, look at the hypotheses in the research studies. If they are in the "null" form—that is, stating that there will be no relationship among the variables—and the research hypothesis is rejected, it supports the theory (Kerlinger, 1986). If the hypothesis is supported, implying no relationship, then it refutes the theory. This sounds confusing, but it is only a function of the way the logic works. Rejecting a null hypothesis is like stating a double negative in English grammar; two "no's" make a "yes." If the hypothesis is not in the null form but actually specifies a relationship, then if the hypothesis is rejected, it refutes the theory and if it is accepted, it supports the theory.

Supporting evidence for a statement must be evaluated quantitatively as well as qualitatively. A brief series of questions is sufficient to give the analyst a general idea of the validity of the research. They are as follows (Kerlinger, 1986):

1. Do the research questions or hypotheses accurately reflect the theoretical concepts?
2. Are the sampling and sample size adequate for the method chosen?
3. Is the methodology sound and appropriate for the questions or hypotheses proposed?
4. Is the data analysis accurate and appropriate?
5. Are the results reported accurately?
6. Are the conclusions justified?
7. Is the study replicable?

If the answers to these questions are satisfactory, the support is sound. However, if one sound study is good as support for a statement, 4 or even 10 sound studies are that much better.

Logical Adequacy

Because this is basically a strategies book, we will not go as far as the linguistic philosophers in determining the logical adequacy of a theory. Linguistic philosophical analysis can get very complicated as it is based on formal logic. We will limit ourselves to only a few considerations: (1) Is there a system whereby predictions can be made from the theory *independent* of its content? (2) Can scientists in the discipline in which the theory is developed agree on those predictions? (3) Does the actual content make sense? (4) Are there obvious logical fallacies?

Predictions Independent of Content   In several previous chapters we have used letters of the alphabet and arrows with pluses or minuses over them to denote symbolically how concepts are related to each other. This is precisely the same kind of system that can be used to determine predictions from a theory that are independent of its content. That is, each of the concepts is given a meaningless label such as *A*, *B*, or *C* and then the relationships are diagrammed, as are the predictions that can be made from those relationships. This step is important when you are concerned with the logical structure of the theory. If the structure is not logical, predicted relationships may be fallacious. This is not to imply that the content itself is unimportant—only that at this time it is not considered. Content

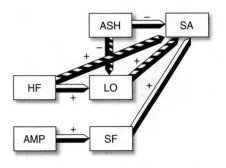

FIGURE 11–1 Diagram of statements 1 through 4 in text.

is analyzed in the meaning steps and also in question 3 in this step. If the theory being analyzed cannot be examined in this way, it leaves much to be desired in terms of logical adequacy. This diagramming effort also points out unclear or unstudied relationships among concepts that are useful for further theory development or research. Below are several relational statements from a theory about the hearing accuracy of a barn owl (Knudsen, 1981).

1. An owl's strike accuracy deteriorates with increases in angle between sound source and head orientation.
2. An owl's ability to locate the origin of a sound is dependent on the presence of high frequencies in the sound.
3. The amount of sound amplification provided by the feathers of the facial ruff varies with the sound frequency.
4. The strike accuracy of the owl increases sharply as the number of frequencies in a sound is increased.

As the original theory is stated, the outcome is strike accuracy. One should be alert to implied relationships. For example, logically the owl must be able to locate the sound source to improve strike accuracy. The statements may be restated as follows:

1. Angle of sound source and head orientation $(ASH) \xrightarrow{-}$ strike accuracy (SA).
2. High frequencies in the sound $(HF) \xrightarrow{+}$ location of origin (LO).
3. Amount of sound amplification $(AMP) \xrightarrow{+}$ sound frequency (SF).
4. Number of sound frequencies $(SF) \xrightarrow{+}$ strike accuracy (SA).

Once they are written and labels assigned, a diagram may be drawn as we have done in Figure 11–1. The relationships that have been specified in the theory are drawn with solid lines. Striped lines indicate the relationships that are implied. All other relationships are unknown.

Now look at Figure 11–2. This is similar to a correlation table, in which all the variables are listed horizontally as well as vertically and the sign of the relationship is placed in the correct box. Implied relationships are enclosed in parenthe-

	SA	LO	AMP	ASH	HF	SF
SA	+	(+)	?	–	(+)	+
LO		+	?	(–)	+	?
AMP			+	?	?	+
ASH				+	?	?
HF					+	?
SF						+

FIGURE 11–2   Another type of matrix showing statements in Figure 11–1.

ses (). As you can see, the matrix is easier to read and the implied relationships can be seen more clearly than in Figure 11–1. Either is acceptable if it helps you get the structure of the relationships clear. If neither is helpful or you feel confused, refer to Chapter 8 on statement analysis for additional help or review.

Agreement of Scientists   A theory must be sufficiently precise in its representation for scientists to agree on the predictions that can be made from it. If scientists cannot agree on the possible predictions, the theory is not useful in any scientific sense. If the theory is not scientifically useful, it cannot be added to any body of knowledge (except, of course, to the body of knowledge of "things that don't work yet"). For an excellent example of how to determine agreement among scientists, see Carter and Kulbok's (1995) evaluation of the Interaction Model of Client Health Behavior.

Making Sense   A theory may make a great deal of sense to one scientist and no sense to another with a different background. For instance, a theory that makes sense to a maternity nurse may make little sense to one in cardiac care. If scientists with relevant and similar backgrounds all say the theory makes no sense, then it probably doesn't. For a theory to make sense, it must provide insights or understanding about a phenomenon. If it does not, perhaps the theorist needs to spend additional time simplifying or more clearly defining what the theory purports to demonstrate in order to meet the criterion of making sense.

Logical Fallacies   Look for logical fallacies. This is where the inductive or deductive origins of the theory become important. In a deductive theory, if all the premises are true and the deduction is valid, then the conclusions, or inferences, drawn from those premises are also true (Toulmin, 1958). Therefore, the analyst must determine whether or not the premises of the theory are true. This usually involves a brief review of literature and an evaluation of any supporting evidence to determine the truth of the premise. In this case truth comes from the validity of the research on which the original premises are based. If the premises are correct, then the conclusion will be also.

In traditional philosophical analysis there are three possible problems with an inductive theory: (1) the premises are correct, but the conclusion is incorrect; (2) the premises are incorrect, but the conclusion is correct; or (3) both premises and conclusion are incorrect (Toulmin, 1958). Again, the analyst must return to the literature and to evidence that supports or refutes the premises. In this case the evidence will be *logically* inconclusive because the theory is inductive. The analyst will simply have to use the notion of the "preponderance of evidence" to determine the relative truth of the premises. If the evidence strongly supports the premises, one can assume truth for the purposes of analysis.

Because the truth of the premises does not guarantee the truth of the conclusion, determining the correctness of the conclusion is more difficult in an inductive theory. All the analyst can do here is examine the research that supports the conclusion for validity and determine if the conclusion makes sense given the stated premises and the research evidence. If the conclusion makes sense and if the research is valid and meets all the criteria for a "good" research study, then the analyst is justified in assuming that the conclusion is correct. If the conclusion fails to make sense or if the research is poor, no assumptions can be made at all about the conclusion. We simply will not know if the conclusion is correct.

In more postmodern philosophy there is less emphasis on the issue of inductive evidence of a theory's validity. Because much of grounded theory, for instance, is generated from inductive and often qualitative research, other criteria for validity are used for the research. For an in-depth discussion of this issue, Sandelowski's article (1986) is excellent. For the purposes of theory analysis either set of criteria will work well to help you evaluate the soundness of the research evidence.

Inductive theory is always logically inconclusive, thus we are always left a bit in doubt about the theory's validity. This doubt does not preclude our use of well-supported theory. It only serves to remind us that there may be a better explanation that has not been discovered yet.

Although the final four steps in theory analysis are not so rigorous or time consuming, they are an important part of a thorough analysis. There are several examples of theory analyses in the literature (Haigh, 2002; Henderson, 1995; Jacono, 1995; Jezewski, 1995; Mitchell, 2001; Olson & Hanchett, 1997; Sigsworth, 1995).

Usefulness

If the theory provides new insights into a phenomenon, if it helps the scientist explain the phenomenon better or differently, or if it helps the scientist make better predictions, then it is a useful theory (Berthold, 1968). It adds significantly to the body of knowledge. If the theory does none of these things it is not a useful theory. Usefulness of theory thus has to do with how helpful the theory is to the scientist in providing a sense of understanding about the phenomenon in question (Reynolds, 1971).

The analyst must consider three issues in determining usefulness: (1) How much research has the theory generated (Reynolds, 1971)? (2) To what clinical problem is the theory relevant (Barnum, 2000)? (3) Does the theory have the potential to influence nursing practice, education, administration, or research (Meleis, 1990)? It is at this point in the analysis that the *content* becomes important. An analyst cannot answer these three questions without considering the content of the theory. If the theory contains subject matter that is already in the scientific domain, it should shed new light on the phenomenon or should provide information that allows clarification, new predictions, or the exertion of control where none previously existed. If the theory covers subject matter that has not been in the scientific domain, it should make some significant difference in that field of science in which it was developed. The theory should generate a significant number of research studies if it is useful. It should be relevant, or at least *potentially* relevant, to a clinical practice setting. It should be capable of influencing, or potentially capable of influencing, nursing practice, education, administration, or research (Meleis, 1990).

Generalizability

How widely the theory can be used in explaining or predicting phenomena reflects the criterion of generalizability or transferability (Lincoln & Guba, 1985). Generalizability can be determined by examining the boundaries of the theory and by evaluating the research that supports the theory. We have said earlier in this chapter that the boundaries of the theory are content related and have to do with how wide the focus of the content is. The wider the focus of a theory, the more generalizable it is likely to be. The more broadly it can be applied, the more generalizable it is. Feminist theorists and critical social theorists use a slightly different set of criteria to evaluate the transferability of a theory. For more detailed discussions of these theories and how they are to be evaluated, we recommend Lincoln and Guba (1985) or Hall and Stevens (1991).

The analyst must have some skills in research critique in order to determine the adequacy of theoretical support because the research evidence that supports the theory is important in determining generalizability. If the research evidence is sound, that is, valid and with adequate sample size, derived from diverse populations, and reproducible, the theory will be more generalizable than one in which there is little support or the research support is of poor quality. It is not our purpose here to provide research critique skills. Any good research textbook can be helpful to the reader who perceives a need for additional help.

Parsimony

A parsimonious theory is one that is elegant in its simplicity even though it may be broad in its content. Perhaps the best example of parsimony is from Einstein's theory of relativity, $E = MC^2$. This particular statement of the theory revolutionized physics and is very broad in its boundaries but is very simple in its expression. A parsimonious theory explains a complex phenomenon simply and briefly without sacrificing the theory's content, structure, or completeness.

Most theories, especially those in the behavioral sciences, cannot be reduced to such a mathematical model. The analyst must examine the theory to see if its formulations are as clear and as brief as they can be. The propositions or relational statements should be precise and should not overlap. If there are several statements, determine if some of them could be reduced to one or two broader, more general, relational statements.

Many theorists provide models as a way of helping themselves and others visualize the relations of the concepts to each other. If such a model is provided, it should accurately reflect the verbal material in the theory. It must also actually help make the theory clearer. If it does not help clarify the verbal material, it is not a useful model and does not aid in increasing the parsimony of the theory.

Testability

We support the idea that for a theory to be truly valid, it must be testable at least in principle. This implies that hypotheses can be generated from the theory, research carried out, and the theory supported by the evidence or modified because of it. A theory that has strong empirical evidence to support it is a stronger theory than one that does not. If a theory cannot generate hypotheses, it is not useful to scientists and does not add to the body of knowledge.

There is some discussion among philosophers of science as to whether or not the criterion of testability is crucial to theory (Hempel, 1965; Popper, 1965; Reynolds, 1971). The debate seems to center on whether or not a theory that provides a great deal of understanding but that by its nature is untestable is a legitimate theory. We do not propose to enter this argument. It seems to us that even a theory that by its nature is untestable as a whole may yield testable hypotheses and relational statements that lend support to the total theory.

ADVANTAGES AND LIMITATIONS

The major advantage of theory analysis is the insight into relationships among the concepts and their linkages to each other that the strategy provides. In addition, the analysis strategy allows the theorist to see the strengths of the theory as well as its weaknesses. The theorist is then free to decide whether or not the theory is useful for practice or research or whether the theory needs additional testing and validation before use. Where a theory has untested linkages discovered through analysis, it is a spur to the theorist to test those linkages. This both strengthens the theory and adds to the body of knowledge. The major limitation of theory analysis is that analysis examines only parts and their relationship to the whole. It can expose only what is missing, but cannot generate new information. In addition, theory analysis requires evaluation and criticism of supporting evidence. Where the analyst may be limited in the critical skills of research evaluation, important information regarding the soundness of a theory may be disregarded or misinterpreted. This results in a limited analysis and may yield unsatisfactory results.

UTILIZING THE RESULTS OF THEORY ANALYSIS

Theory analysis provides a means of systematic examination of the structure and content of theory for new insights into a phenomenon or to determine its strengths and weaknesses. But what does one do with the analysis when it is completed? The results of theory analysis can be very useful in education, practice, research, and theory development.

Theory analysis can be used very effectively in the classroom. We have used it successfully to teach students how to examine theories critically. Assigning a theory to a group of students to analyze and then having them report to the class often generates meaningful discussion and debate among the students. Another use of the results of theory analysis is in preparing conceptual frameworks for students' papers. Students have found theory analysis an excellent way to define gaps or inconsistencies in the knowledge about some phenomenon in which they are interested. Yet a third use of the results of theory analysis is in faculty development. As we proposed in the statement analysis chapter, having faculty discussions related to the results of theory analysis on a single topic of interest may generate many useful ideas to be used in curriculum design or in generating faculty research.

The results of theory analysis may provide the clinician with knowledge about the soundness of any theory being considered for adoption in practice. In addition, knowing which theoretical relationships are well supported provides guidelines for the choice of appropriate interventions and some indications of their efficacy. Given the current emphasis on evidence-based practice, the results of theory analysis will assist clinicians to determine whether or not a particular theory might be appropriate for their practice.

Theory analysis is particularly helpful in research because it provides a clear idea of the form and structure of the theory in addition to the relevance of content, and inconsistencies and gaps present. The "missing links" or inconsistencies are fruitful sources of new research ideas. They also point to the next hypotheses that need to be tested. In theory development, the inconsistencies, gaps, and missing links provide the stimulus to the theorist to keep on working. In addition, the results provide clues to the obvious next steps to be taken to refine the theory.

SUMMARY

Theory analysis consists of systematically examining a theory for its origins, meaning, logical adequacy, usefulness, generalizability/parsimony, and testability. Each of these six steps stands alone in a theory analysis and yet each is related to the other. This paradoxical relationship is generated by the act of analysis itself. To do a thorough analysis, one must consider each of the steps, giving them all careful attention. Yet, the results of each of the steps are interdependent on the results of the others.

Like many of the strategies presented in this book, the steps of theory analysis are also iterative. That is, the analyst must go back and forth among the steps during the analysis in addition to moving sequentially through them.

For instance, the logical adequacy, usefulness, generalizability, parsimony, and testability of a theory will be affected if concepts are undefined and statements are only definitional in nature. If the meaning is adequately handled but the logical structure is missing or fallacious, then usefulness, generalizability, parsimony, and testability will be severely limited. If a theory is untestable and fails to generate hypotheses, it is not useful, generalizable, parsimonious, or particularly meaningful. So each step is independent and yet interdependent as well. It is this interdependence that makes the strategy so useful in theory construction. The analysis strategy provides a mechanism for determining the strengths and weaknesses of the theory prior to using it as a guide to practice or in research.

With theory analysis, linkages that have not been examined become obvious. This, in turn, should lead to additional testing, thus adding support to the theory or pointing out where modifications need to be made. The whole process is complex but the results are well worth the effort. It frequently leads to new insights about the theory being examined, thus adding to the body of knowledge.

Theory analysis, like all analysis strategies, is rigorous and takes time. It is also limited in that it does not generate new information outside the confines of the theory.

Finally, by pointing out where additional theoretical work is needed, theory analysis is a way of promoting additional theory construction. When pointing out where additional work is needed, however, it is helpful to remember that comparing anything to the ideal tends to stifle development (Zetterberg, 1965). The best approach is to compare the analyzed theory to similar theories at the same stage of development. To what extent does this theory meet the criteria as compared to others similar to it? Because most theories are generated in the context of discovery, it is more helpful to be encouraging than to be severely critical.

PRACTICE EXERCISE

Read Younger's (1991) "A Theory of Mastery." It is a relatively new theory and is substantially middle range in focus. It is therefore suitable to use for your practice exercise.

Conduct a theory analysis. When you have completed your own analysis, compare it to the one below. Keep in mind that your analysis will probably be more comprehensive than the one we have included here. Our intention is to give you only clues as to the major strengths and weaknesses of the theory. The example we have provided is merely a sample to demonstrate each step. Remember that although one person's analysis may differ somewhat from another's, they may both be equally valid.

Origins

Younger developed the theory of mastery in an effort to explain "how individuals who experience illness or other stressful health conditions and enter into a state of stress may emerge, not demoralized and vulnerable, but healthy and possibly stronger" (p. 77). In addition, she states that a second purpose was to explicate the theory base for the new instrument she is developing. The theory appears to be a deductive synthesis based on various philosophical and empirical works of others, but Younger is not explicit about whether it is a deductive system.

Meaning

1. The major concepts identified by Younger in addition to mastery are

   certainty
   change
   acceptance
   growth

   In addition to the five major concepts, Younger mentions several related concepts. These are coping, adjustment, efficacy, resilience, hardiness, and control. In each case, she attempts to identify how the related concepts are different from mastery.
   Not identified as a part of the theory or related concepts but discussed in the section on the definition of mastery are such concepts as quality of life, bonds of connectedness with others, stress, self-curing, self-caring, hypervigilance, compulsive repetition, sleep disturbance, fearfulness, passivity, and alienation. These concepts are part of the discussions about antecedents and consequences of mastery or the lack of achievement of mastery.

2. The major concepts—certainty, change, acceptance, growth, and mastery—are all carefully defined. Indeed, it appears from the discussion that all five have been subjected to concept analysis. As a result, these five concepts have excellent descriptive and theoretical definitions that are used consistently throughout the piece. There are no operational definitions given here. However, it appears that these may be forthcoming as one of the purposes of the article was to give a theory base for a new instrument.

3. The relational statements are harder to come by in this work than are the concepts. Each concept in the theory is described as a process that must be completed before mastery can be achieved. Below are the statements Younger makes explicitly about the relationships among the concepts:

   a. A critical dose of certainty is necessary for change and acceptance.
   b. Change and acceptance are necessary for growth to occur.
   c. Change, acceptance, and growth feed back to increase certainty.
   d. Change is sufficient for growth.
   e. Change and acceptance are dynamically interrelated.

   f.   Acceptance, qualified, is sufficient for growth.
   g.   Stress initiates the process of mastery.
   h.   Mastery affects quality of life and wellness.

   Each of the statements indicates a positive relationship. The boundaries
   are moderately wide. The theory is abstract but is sufficiently circum-
   scribed to be considered a middle-range theory.
      The statements are all made toward the end of the article and are not
   used again once they are made. Therefore, no judgment can be made about
   the degree to which the author uses them consistently. One must look to
   later works to make this judgment.
      There is no empirical support given for any of the statements. There
   is some philosophical and historical background given as justification for
   them but no testing has been done as yet using this new theory.

Logical Adequacy

   1. It is possible to make predictions independent of content. The matrix
      shown in Figure 11–3 demonstrates where the predictions are specified
      and where they are implied. Some of the major concepts of the theory are
      included here, although there are several other relevant concepts men-
      tioned in the narrative.

      certainty (CT)   acceptance (A)
      stress (S)   wellness (W)
      change (CG)   growth (G)
      quality of life (QOL)

	CT	CG	A	G	S	QOL	W
CT	+	+	+	+	(–)	(+)	(+)
CG		+	+	+	(–)	(–)	(–)
A			+	+	(–)	(+)	(+)
G				+	(–)	(+)	(+)
S					+	(–)	(–)
QOL						+	(+)
W							+

FIGURE 11–3   Matrix of concepts in theory of mastery.

Obviously there are many implied, but unspecified relationships in the theory. Some of the implied relationships are supported in other research in the field but are not indicated in Younger's article.

2. The theory is relatively new and so agreement of scientists is probable but not confirmed by the use of the theory in others' work to date. However, it seems reasonable that such agreement is possible. Although the theory is still untested, it is capable of test. Therefore, this criterion is met in principle but not in fact.

3. The theory makes sense as it is built on several sound philosophical and scientific traditions. It is appealing in its simplicity. However, it is a bit redundant of other similar theories. It is very close indeed to various theories of self-efficacy for instance.

4. There are no logical fallacies, although there are some logical relationships that as yet go unspecified and are only implied in the theory.

Usefulness

The theory has the potential to be useful. Even though it is somewhat similar to other theories of coping and self-efficacy, it is specifically focused on threats to health as a primary stressor. For this reason alone it may prove very helpful to practitioners and researchers in nursing.

Generalizability or Transferability

The theory has relatively wide boundaries, but so far has not been tested or verified through research. Certainly it would apply to anyone experiencing stress, particularly health-related stress. Its potential for explanatory power is excellent.

Parsimony

The theory is relatively new and therefore is probably too parsimonious. It seems that there is a natural evolution or progression of new theories such that they often start small and parsimonious, grow substantially during the justification phases, and then are reduced to smaller and more parsimonious models over time. This theory is still very new. It may undergo substantial changes and revisions before it is considered to be adequately developed.

Testability

Given appropriate, reliable, and valid instruments to measure the concepts in this theory *as they are defined,* the theory is testable. The concepts are very carefully defined, so any instruments being considered for testing them should be examined carefully to be sure that they reflect the defining attributes of each of the concepts.

REFERENCES

Barnum B. *Nursing Theory: Analysis, Application, and Evaluation.* 5th ed. Philadelphia, Penn: Lippincott; 2000.

Berthold FS. Symposium on theory development in nursing. *Nurs Res.* 1968;17(3):196-197.

Carter KF, Kulbok PA. Evaluation of the Interaction Model of Client Health Behavior through the first decade of research. *Adv Nurs Sci.* 1995;18(1):62-73.

Chinn P, Jacobs M. *Theory and Nursing: A Systematic Approach.* 2nd ed. St. Louis, Mo: Mosby; 1987.

Cooley ME. Analysis and evaluation of the Trajectory Theory of Chronic Illness Management. *Scholar Inquiry Nurs Pract.* 1999;13(2):75-95.

Dickoff J, James P, Wiedenbach E. Theory in a practice discipline, part I. *Nurs Res.* 1968a;17:415-435.

Dickoff J, James P, Wiedenbach E. Theory in a practice discipline, part II. *Nurs Res.* 1968b; 17:545-554.

Fawcett J. A framework for analysis and evaluation of conceptual models of nursing. *Nurs Educ.* 1980;5(6):10-14.

Fawcett J. *Analysis and Evaluation of Conceptual Models of Nursing.* 2nd ed. Philadelphia, Penn: Davis; 1989.

Fawcett J. *Analysis and Evaluation of Conceptual Models of Nursing.* 3rd ed. Philadelphia, Penn: Davis; 1995.

Fawcett J. *Analysis and Evaluation of Contemporary Nursing Knowledge: Nursing Models and Theories.* Philadelphia, Penn: Davis; 2000.

Fawcett J. *Analysis and Evaluation of Nursing Theories.* Philadelphia, Penn: Davis; 1993.

Hage J. *Techniques and Problems of Theory Construction in Sociology.* New York, NY: Wiley; 1972.

Haigh C. Using chaos theory: the implication for nursing. *J Adv Nurs.* 2002;37(5):462-469.

Hall JM, Stevens PE. Rigor in feminist research. *Adv Nurs Sci.* 1991;13(3):16-29.

Hardy M. Theories: components, development, evaluation. *Nurs Res.* 1974;23(2):100-106.

Hempel CG. *Aspects of Scientific Explanation.* New York, NY: Free Press; 1965.

Hempel CG. *Philosophy of Natural Science.* Englewood Cliffs, NJ: Prentice Hall; 1966.

Henderson DJ. Consciousness raising in participatory research: method and methodology for emancipatory nursing inquiry. *Adv Nurs Sci.* 1995;17(3):58-69.

Jacono BJ. A holistic exploration of barriers to theory utilization. *J Adv Nurs.* 1995; 21(3):515-519.

Jezewski MA. Evolution of a grounded theory: conflict resolution through culture brokering. *Adv Nurs Sci.* 1995;17(3):14-30.

Kerlinger F. *Foundations of Behavioral Research.* 3rd ed. New York, NY: Holt, Rinehart & Winston; 1986.

Knudsen EL. The hearing of the barn owl. *Sci Am.* 1981;245(6):113-125.

Lincoln YS, Guba EQ. *Naturalistic Inquiry.* Beverly Hills, Calif: Sage Publications; 1985.

Meleis A. *Theoretical Nursing: Development and Progress.* Philadelphia, Penn: Lippincott; 1990.

Mitchell G. Prescription, freedom, and participation: drilling down into theory-based nursing practice. *Nurs Sci Q.* 2001;14(3):205-210.

Olson J, Hanchett J. Nurse-expressed empathy, patient outcomes, and development of a middle-range theory. *Image.* 1997;29(1):71-76.

Popper KR. *Conjectures and Refutations: The Growth of Scientific Knowledge.* New York, NY: Harper & Row; 1965.

Popper KR. *The Logic of Scientific Discovery.* New York, NY: Science Editions; 1961.

Reynolds PD. *A Primer in Theory Construction.* Indianapolis, Ind: Bobbs-Merrill; 1971.

Sandelowski M. The problem of rigor in qualitative research. *Adv Nurs Sci.* 1986;8(3):27-37.

Sigsworth J. Feminist research: its relevance to nursing. *J Adv Nurs* 1995;22(5):896-899.

Toulmin S. *The Uses of Argument.* London, England: Cambridge University Press; 1958.

Wilson J. *Thinking with Concepts.* New York, NY: Cambridge University Press; 1969.

Younger JB. A theory of mastery. *Adv Nurs Sci.* 1991;14(1):76-89.

Zetterberg HL. *On Theory and Verification in Sociology.* Totowa, NJ: Bedminster Press; 1965.

ADDITIONAL READINGS

Aldous J. Strategies for developing family theory. *J Marriage Fam.* 1970;32:250-257.

Blalock HM. *Theory Construction: From Verbal to Mathematical Formulations.* Englewood Cliffs, NJ: Prentice Hall; 1969.

Copi I. *Introduction to Logic.* 7th ed. New York, NY: Macmillan; 1986.

Hanson NR. *Patterns of Discovery.* London, England: Cambridge University Press; 1958.

Hutchinson SA, Wilson HS. The theory of unpleasant symptoms and Alzheimer's disease. *Scholar Inquiry Nurs Pract.* 1998;12(2):143-158.

Kaplan A. *The Conduct of Inquiry.* New York, NY: Chandler; 1964.

Lenz ER, Gift AG. Response to "the theory of unpleasant symptoms and Alzheimer's disease." *Scholar Inquiry Nurs Pract.* 1998;12(2):159-162.

Lenz ER, Pugh LC, Milligan RA, Gift A, Suppe F. The middle-range theory of unpleasant symptoms: an update. *Adv Nurs Sci.* 1997;19(3):14-27.

Lenz ER, Suppe F, Gift F, Pugh LC, Milligan RA. Collaborative development of middle-range nursing theories: toward a theory of unpleasant symptoms. *Adv Nurs Sci.* 1995; 17(3):1-13.

Paley J. Benner's remnants: culture, tradition and everyday understanding. *J Adv Nurs.* 2002;38(6):566–573.

Roberson MR, Kelley JH. Using Orem's theory in transcultural settings: a critique. *Nurs Forum.* 1996;31(3):22-28.

Silva MC. Response to "analysis and evaluation of the trajectory theory of chronic illness management." *Scholar Inquiry Nurs Pract.* 1999;13(2):96-109.

PART V

Perspectives on Nursing Theory

In this final part of the book, we step back and broaden our view. Our goal is to put the specifics of theory development into context. First, Chapter 12 focuses on concept, statement, and theory testing (validation), an idea briefly introduced in Chapter 2. This is an important and often neglected activity in evolving the theoretical basis for the nursing discipline. Theory testing involves logical operations and empirical research, both of which are briefly addressed in Chapter 12.

In Chapter 13 we present two topics that stand out as rapidly developing areas of scholarship related to theory development in recent literature. We call them frontiers of theory development. The first topic is progress in international and ethnicity-related nursing theory development. Many nurses think of theory development only in terms of scholarship emanating from the United States. Even though our sources are limited to English-language articles, the literature reviewed for this chapter makes it clear that theory development in nursing is a worldwide phenomenon and in the United States reaches beyond the dominant culture.

The second topic consists of the tandem areas of nursing informatics and evidence-based practice. As research emphasis shifted toward evidence-based practice, so did the discussions of what impact it might have on theory development. Simultaneously, the emphasis increased on documentation of nursing care to provide the needed evidence.

12

Concept, Statement, and Theory Testing

Preliminary Note: *Shifting gears from theory development to theory testing (or from the context of discovery to justification) can be both exhilarating and trying. Readers should be aware that they may experience a feeling of being at sea. Some of the intellectual freedom of movement that can be so useful in the development process may be replaced by a desire for greater direction and clarity about testing methodology. Despite having taken research methods courses, the specific methods of concept, statement, and theory testing may not be easily extracted from those didactic experiences. Thus, in this chapter, we have aimed at providing an intellectual bridge between research methods and testing the fruits of concept, statement, and theory development. Because these intellectual products may vary widely, there is no one method that can be applied to all cases. As always, judgment is involved.*

INTRODUCTION

The 11 chapters preceding this one have covered the context, terminology, and strategies of theory development. In this chapter we shift our emphasis to the vital next phase that follows the initial development of concepts, statements, and theory. (Note that we use *testing* in a broad, not restrictive, sense. For the most part, *testing* and *empirical validation* are equivalent terms. *Testing* is a more familiar term, however, to many readers.) In Chapter 2, we presented a model of the phases in the development of nursing science (see Figure 2–2). The first phases depicted in that model include developing concepts, statements, and theories in nursing. The subsequent phases of development, testing, revision, and retesting portrayed in our model demonstrate the necessary and reciprocal links between the contexts of discovery and justification in building nursing science. Along this line, the noted methodologist Marx (1963) observed the following:

> We need to recognize most explicitly that both *discovery* and *confirmation* are necessary to effective scientific work. The most ingenious theories are limited [sic] value

until empirical tests are produced; the best confirmed proposition is of little value unless it deals with meaningful variables. (p. 13)

In this chapter we assume that the concept, statement, or theory that has been the focus of a theorist's developmental activities is of sufficient import to warrant testing. This assumption serves as our point of departure for now considering testing of concepts, statements, and theories.

As we turn to the topic of concept, statement, and theory testing, it is important to note that this topic is embedded in diverse philosophical issues that have arisen about the nature of science and the varieties (and relevance) of scientific knowledge and methodologies. Some of these have been briefly profiled in Chapter 1. Although exposition of such issues is not possible here, interested readers may find the following sources useful: Coward (1990) on worldviews of scientific inquiry; Holter (1988) on philosophical orientations to nursing theory; Schumacher and Gortner (1992) on misconceptions in nursing about traditional science; and Silva and Sorrell (1992) on alternative approaches (critical reasoning, personal experience, and application to practice) to testing nursing theories. Fuller review of many of these issues is provided by Phillips (1987) and Fiske and Shweder (1986). In this chapter, our presentation of concept, statement, and theory testing is concerned primarily with empirical validity.

CONCEPT TESTING

Concepts often are the focal point of theoretic activity because they are critical in delineating problems or phenomena in clinical practice. Concepts such as insufficient milk supply (Hill & Humenick, 1989), chronic fatigue (Potempa, Lopez, Reid, & Lawson, 1986), and chronic dyspnea (McCarley, 1999) are among those that have been of interest to nurses. Whether concepts originate from synthesis of observations, derivation from other fields, analysis of existing ideas, or still other methods, it is often necessary to empirically validate the existence and clinical relevance of the concept and its purported properties. Even if a concept is embedded in a loose network of related concepts, it is sometimes useful to focus first on the empirical validation of that concept, especially if it is critical to developing a continuing program of research.

Empirical validation of concepts is guided by three questions: (1) Is there evidence, and if so how strong is it, that the concept represents a phenomenon in reality? (2) What evidence is there that the concept is relevant to practice, in terms of client needs, clinical outcomes, or other meaningful clinical criteria? (3) What evidence supports the purported attributes of the concept (Pedhazur & Schmelkin call these "reflective indicators" [1991, p. 54])? Gathering the evidence to answer these questions and weighing that evidence as it supports or fails to support the credibility, relevance, and clarity of the concept is not a black-and-white or one-time matter. That is, new evidence may call into question earlier judgments. Further, by their very nature these three questions are directed at concepts in general and, thus, may not be well suited to every type of concept. User discretion is advised!

First, a working definition of a concept is required in order to determine whether there is evidence that the concept represents a phenomenon in reality. If possible, the definition should specify conceptual attributes of the concept as well as operational ones so instances of the concept can be identified. This definition can then be used to search the literature for supportive evidence as well as to design concept validation studies (see Waltz, Strickland, & Lenz [1991] for a model of how to operationalize concepts and Pedhazur & Schmelkin [1991] on construct validation).

A historical example illustrates better than directives what is involved in validating a concept. Klaus and Kennell (1976) and Klaus et al. (1972) proposed that the concept of attachment or bonding may apply to humans as it does to animals. In animals, they noted that separation of mother and offspring immediately after birth was associated with "deviant behavior" (Klaus et al., 1972, p. 460). What was unknown was whether the "bonding" concept represented a phenomenon that also occurred in human mothers. By providing an opportunity for extended contact shortly after birth—their operational definition of the conditions necessary for attachment or bonding to occur—Klaus et al. tested for the existence of attachment in human mothers. In later noting that mothers who had extra contact responded differently to their infants, they took that evidence to support a concept of human mother–infant bonding (Klaus & Kennell, 1976). As additional evidence accumulated and was evaluated critically by others, however, Klaus and Kennell (1982) watered down their claims about the existence of animal-type bonding in humans. Thus, the credibility of the original Klaus and Kennell bonding concept has decreased as additional evidence has been inconsistent or as that evidence has been judged to be flawed in nature.

Second, even if a concept appears to represent some phenomenon in reality, such existence does not in itself render the concept of high relevance to practice. That is, there must also be some reason to believe that the introduction of the concept into scientific discourse can aid in meeting—at some level—the practice aims of the nursing discipline. One might ask (1) what client needs a concept addresses, (2) what guidance the concept gives to the content of nursing actions, or (3) what clinical outcomes are clarified or enhanced by virtue of the insight provided by the concept? Evidence of relevance to practice may come from many sources. These include, but are not limited to, existing literature that identifies problems needing conceptual solutions, opinions of expert clinicians in the area the concept has relevance to, and perceptions of nursing clients. For example, the concept of bonding had high practice relevance based on consumer interest in it. According to McCall (1987), "The general public was . . . ready to hear the good news, because the apparent benefits of early contact fit nicely with the movement toward more humane birthing practices" (p. 1229). On the other hand, Billings (1995) has argued more recently that the uncritical application of bonding theory in practice could be oppressive to women.

Third, evidence related to attributes of a concept clarifies the dimensions, components, or other features that are essential to that concept (see Chapter 5 on defining attributes of concepts). Procedures and methods for testing attributes of a concept have been extensively developed in relation to the areas of tests and measurement (see Pedhazur & Schmelkin, 1991; Waltz et al., 1991) and nursing diagnosis and intervention development and validation (see Avant, 1979; Fehring, 1986; Gordon & Sweeney, 1979; McCloskey & Bulechek, 2000). Refer to those respective literatures for in-depth treatment of attribute validation. Our intent here is to give general guidelines for concept-attribute testing.

To facilitate concept testing, the theorist should specify in advance (1) whether the purported attributes are all equally central to the concept and (2) whether there is a hierarchical structure to attributes. By making a clear proposal about concept attributes it is easier to interpret the results of testing. Further, testing and interpretation of results can be done with greater clarity if the theorist specifies the likely antecedents of the concept (called "formative indicators" by Pedhazur & Schmelkin [1991, p. 54]) in contrast to its defining attributes (Pedhazur & Schmelkin's reflective indicators). Stating in advance what are the boundaries of a concept and its attributes with respect to specific client populations is also helpful. Wide generalizability makes a concept more useful. However, careful testing with delimited populations can aid in differentiating between a concept with poorly identified attributes versus inconsistencies in concept manifestations stemming from different populations. Subsequently, areas of difference in attributes can be tested in new groups (e.g., see Fry & Nguyen's [1996] test of the symptoms of depression in Australian and Vietnamese groups).

Attribute testing may take many forms. One of the most common is generating items that reflect discrete instances of the various attributes of a concept and subsequently analyzing these items through statistical procedures such as factor analysis. Such analysis aids in determining if purported attributes indeed can be demonstrated empirically. In many respects the processes of concept testing and instrument development overlap. For some practice-based concepts, such as confusion (Nagley & Byers, 1987), more clinically relevant methods of testing are needed. Nagley and Byers have proposed the idea of clinical construct validity wherein "a test reflects the clinical correlates that comprise a phenomenon as viewed from the nursing perspective in nursing situations" (p. 619). For an example of testing defining attributes in the context of nursing diagnosis, see Carlson-Catalano et al., (1998).

Finally, despite the fact that we have treated concept, statement, and theory testing separately to distinguish among each type of testing, frequently there is overlap among them. Often a concept is the focal point for theoretic work, but the concept itself may be seen by the theorist as occurring within a network of other concepts. For example, the concepts of insufficient milk supply (Hill & Humenick, 1989) and chronic fatigue (Potempa, Lopez, Reid, & Lawson, 1986) mentioned earlier both are located within models that depict their relationships to other concepts. The stage of evolution of a program of scholarship determines whether it is more useful to approach testing as concept-, statement-, or theory-focused.

STATEMENT TESTING

Testing the empirical validity of statements is probably the form of testing with which readers are most familiar. Research texts (see Polit & Beck, 2003) typically present hypotheses to be tested as statements of relationships between two or more variables. Depending on the nature of the concepts linked in statements, those statements usually are tested in descriptive–correlational or experimental designs. Refer to extant research texts for guidance in designing and conducting hypothesis-testing research.

The measures of concepts should be selected with great care in testing statements. If a measure is not a good reflective indicator (Pedhazur & Schmelkin, 1991) of a concept, misleading inferences can be made about the credibility of the statement put to test. Furthermore, judgments about the credibility of statements depend on the quantity and quality of accumulated evidence. As a result, not one study but the accumulated evidence across studies is usually considered in determining the credibility of a statement. For example, Susser (1991) carefully weighed the thoroughness and quality of evidence about the causal relationship between maternal nutrition and infant birth weight as mediated by maternal weight gain. Among the conclusions of that rigorous review were the following: "Prenatal diet affects birth weight most, as it does maternal weight, in the third trimester in women starving and acutely hungry. . . . Effects are otherwise more modest and conditional" (p. 1394). Credibility of a statement may change, however, especially if new, high-quality evidence is inconsistent with evidence available previously. What constitutes high-quality evidence may vary, though, with the statement being tested. For example, randomized clinical trials may be appropriate for testing statements about the efficacy of clinical interventions, but be ill-suited for testing predictive statements about health disparities of groups.

Keep in mind that there is not always a hard-and-fast line between concept, statement, and theory testing. For example, although a theory may be tested as a whole in some cases, it is often more feasible to test selected statements from a theory. Thus, statement testing may be part of a larger theory testing enterprise. As a result, many of the concerns identified in the next section on theory testing also can apply to testing theoretically derived statements.

THEORY TESTING

Theory-testing research has been conducted in diverse nursing contexts: preventive care of women (Ehrenberger, Alligood, Thomas, Wallace, & Licavoli, 2002) and men (Nivens, Herman, Weinrich, & Weinrich, 2001); children's (Yeh, 2002) and elder's health (Zauszniewski, Chung, & Krafcik, 2001); chronic illness care related to cancer (Berger & Walker, 2001), HIV (Bova, 2001), and heart disease (Beckie, Beckstead, & Webb, 2001); nursing performance (Doran, Sidani, Keatings, & Doidge, 2002); ethnically diverse populations (Jennings-Dozier, 1999; Villarruel, 1995; Villarruel & Denyes, 1997); various countries (Demerouti, Bakker, Nachreiner, & Schaufeli, 2000; Frey, Rooke, Sieloff, Messmer, & Kameoka, 1995) and geographic communities (McCullagh, Lusk, & Ronis, 2002). Given its ubiquitous nature, it is important to understand this important dimension of nursing knowledge validation.

Theory testing is challenging because of the greater complexity of relationships inherent in theories compared to statements (for example, see Figure 9–1). Furthermore, assessing the empirical validity of a theory has been hampered by lack of clarity about what constitutes sound theory-testing research. Consequently, Silva (1986) proposed seven evaluation criteria that studies aimed at testing conceptual models (grand theories) should ideally meet. Her work is particularly important because it has provided methodological reference points that have been missing from most previous literature on theory testing. Thus, our understanding of what constitutes adequate theory testing was sharpened by her work. Because the concern in this section is with testing a wide variety of middle-range theories that may inform us about nursing phenomena, we have adapted Silva's criteria to fit this more specific application:

1. The purpose of the study is to determine the empirical validity of a designated theory's assumptions or propositions (internal theoretical statements).
2. The theory is explicitly stated as the rationale for the research.
3. The theory's internal structure (key propositions and their interrelationships) is explicitly stated so that its relationship to study hypotheses is clear.
4. The study hypotheses are clearly deduced from the theory's assumptions or propositions.
5. The study hypotheses are empirically tested in an appropriate research design using sound and relevant instruments and suitable study participants.
6. As a result of the empirical testing, evidence exists of the validity or invalidity of the designated assumptions or propositions of the theory.
7. This evidence is considered specifically as it supports, refutes, or explains relevant aspects of the theory.

Even these criteria are lacking in one regard, though. Consider that it is conceivable that hypotheses derived from a theory are compatible with it as well as several other theories and, additionally, that the hypotheses are consistently shown to be congruent with empirical observations. For example, the hypothesis that the poor will experience more health problems than the wealthy is compatible with several theoretical models. Similarly, predicting on theoretical grounds that patients receiving individualized nursing intervention will demonstrate more skill in self-care than those receiving routine care may be derivable from a number of theories. Further, testing a hypothesis such as either of the above carries a low risk for any theories from which they are derived because they would be expected to be supported by the data. Indeed both of the examples given are vague hypotheses that would be difficult to reject. Thus, theory testing is more complex than simply deriving hypotheses and testing them. Not only must researchers be able to derive hypotheses, but they should do so in a way that puts a theory at high risk for falsification (Popper, 1965).

To be falsifiable, a theory must be able to predict with enough specificity that empirical results that are incompatible with the theory can be derived clearly (Fawcett, 1999, p. 95). Wallace (1971) presented an example of this principle in operation.

> *For a simple example, the hypothesis that "all human groups are either stratified or not stratified" is untestable in principle because it does not rule out any logically possible empirical findings. The hypothesis that "all human groups are stratified," however, is testable because it asserts that the discovery of an unstratified human group, though logically possible, will not in fact occur. (p. 78)*

To repeat an old saw: a theory that predicts everything predicts nothing. Or, in the words of Popper, "Every 'good' scientific theory is a prohibition: it forbids certain things to happen. The more a theory forbids, the better it is" (1965, p. 36). Thus, we add still another criterion for theory testing:

8. The hypotheses used to test a specific theory are designed to put the theory at risk for falsification by virtue of their specificity and compatibility with only a limited set of events.

Consistent with this last criterion, the more specific the predictions are that can be made from a theory, the more readily it can be falsified and the narrower the range of data that will support the theory. In testing theories, the theorist must judge how well the results of testing fit with the theories. As theoretical predictions increase in precision, the judgment about "fit" becomes less ambiguous and less arbitrary (Blalock, 1979). Further, if the results of testing highly specific hypotheses result in data that are very consistent with predictions, the theory is judged to be both falsifiable and empirically valid. Consider the following examples. The prediction that "A is associated with B" is less specific than the prediction that "in every case of B, it is preceded by the occurrence of A." As hypotheses formulated in nursing research move increasingly from the former type to the latter, the falsifiability of theories will increase.

Another dimension complicating theory testing is each assumption made in designing testing conditions (Hempel, 1966, pp. 19–32). These assumptions include a wide range of explicit and implicit beliefs such as (1) adequate reliability and validity of measurement procedures used, (2) absence of contaminating circumstances during data collection, and (3) accuracy of any scientific "facts" assumed to be true in designing the research procedures. When results support a theory, the theorist erroneously may have discounted an alternate explanation of the results. Conversely, when results do not support a theoretical prediction, an error may lie not in the theory itself but in the testing conditions. Thus, no one test will definitively refute or substantiate a theory. Theory testing is rather the weight of *accumulated* testing results in varied researches.

Replication of research that tests a promising theory is consequently a strategic aspect in building nursing science. Consequently, empirical validity is a conditional quality of theories; it is tied to the existing evidence pertinent to the theory. As further research is done, a theory that was judged empirically valid at one time may be considered less valid at a later time. Thus, as additional tests of a theory provide evidence that is compatible or incompatible with theoretical predictions, empirical validity grows or shrinks respectively.

Johnson, Ratner, Bottorff, and Hayduk's (1993) study illustrates many facets of the theory-testing process. One of the explicit purposes of their study was to test Pender's (1987) health promotion model (HPM). The HPM specifies that two sets of factors (modifying factors and cognitive–perceptual factors) and cues to action influence the likelihood of health-promoting behaviors. Johnson et al. (1993) noted that the HPM was "well suited" for testing using advanced statistical methods (structural equation models) "because the HPM is composed of clearly specified causal paths" (p. 133). They stated further that "The ordering of the concepts is clear, with 'modifying' or background factors having a causal impact on seven cognitive–perceptual factors that, in turn, affect participation in particular health-promoting behaviors." Thus, demographic characteristics such as age and biological characteristics such as weight indirectly influence health promotion behaviors by modifying cognitive–perceptual factors.

Seven categories of cognitive–perceptual factors directly influence health promotion behaviors. Johnson et al. (1993) focused on three of these: perceived control of health, perceived self-efficacy, and perceived health status. Of five modifying factors, Johnson and colleagues focused on two: demographic characteristics and biological characteristics. Structural equation modeling was used as the data analytic method because it is "the only means by which a simultaneous test of multiple variables can be accomplished" (p. 132). Although they used a delimited set of variables in their test of the HPM, they argued that the components they selected "must fit the data if the overall model is to succeed" (p. 133). Tests of the HPM were carried out using already existing data from a national health survey of over 1,000 adults. Most variables in the test of the HPM were measured by single-item indicators.

Johnson et al. (1993) reported that the implied covariance matrix based on the HPM "differed significantly from the observed covariance matrix, and that the model failed to explain observed relationships" (p. 136). In examining the data for discrepancy from expectations, the investigators noted that, contrary to the HPM, modifying factors exerted direct effects on health promotion behaviors. Finally, the investigators concluded that "The causal structure of the HPM must be reconsidered with a view to fully specifying all of the key factors that affect health-promoting lifestyle and their interrelationships" (p. 138).

The discrepant findings reported by Johnson et al. (1993) point to the final problem faced by the theorist and researcher. It is often easier to cling to a familiar and cherished theory than to abandon it. Although "facts" may seem irrefutable, their interpretation certainly may be influenced by subjective factors. For this reason, we advocate that theory testing be executed, where possible, using multiple competing hypotheses (Platt, 1964). To do this requires that a researcher derive research hypotheses about a phenomenon from several theories and design research to test concurrently each of these. Simultaneously proposing and testing several competing theoretically based hypotheses for their fit and scientific utility reduces the danger that a researcher will be overly wedded to any one theory. Proposing hypotheses from several competing theories and then simultaneously testing these has the added advantage of accelerating the scientific process. Rather than testing one theory, finding it equivocal, and then moving on to testing another, this entire sequence can be merged into one research effort.

One cautionary note must be made with regard to theory testing. Powerful statistical methods, such as structural equation modeling, now exist to test the fit of a model with available data (Tabachnick & Fidell, 2001). Through model modification it is possible to achieve successively better fits of a model with the data. Data-derived model modifications, however, shift the context from justification to discovery. In other words, using the data to simultaneously test and then rebuild and retest a model undermines the credibility of theory testing. Such work should be considered developmental.

Finally, although it is customary to associate theory testing with quantitative methods, such a view is too restrictive. Qualitative methods adapted to the context of justification may also be suited to theory testing.

CONCLUSION

As we pointed out in the first chapter of this book, nursing has generated theory at many levels. Only theory that is sufficiently refined and proposes measurable models of reality, however, is amenable to rigorous testing. Well-articulated theories decrease the arbitrariness of judgments about their merits. This is especially important if a theory base is used in defining directions for policy and practice. Testability of a theory and its empirical validity are of equal or greater importance in nursing as a practice discipline than to basic sciences. The public trust in a profession warrants using the very best procedures in making scientific judgments that have human import.

Interdependence of theory development and testing is essential if nursing is to build a sound body of knowledge for practice. Sustained and diversified development of the theoretic base of nursing practice requires that nurses manifest not only energy and thought in their work, but also long-term commitment. Such commitment is clear when scholarly projects of nurses can be organized into programs of scholarship. For graduate students, it is useful to begin defining that program of scholarship early and framing its possible evolution into the future.

REFERENCES

Avant K. Nursing diagnosis: maternal attachment. *Adv Nurs Sci.* 1979;2(1):45-55.
Beckie TM, Beckstead JW, Webb MS. Modeling women's quality of life after cardiac events. *West J Nurs Res.* 2001;23:179-194.
Berger AM, Walker SN. An explanatory model of fatigue in women receiving adjuvant breast cancer chemotherapy. *Nurs Res.* 2001;50:42-52.
Billings JR. Bonding theory—tying mothers in knots? a critical review of the application of a theory to nursing. *J Clin Nurs.* 1995;4:207-211.
Blalock HM. Dilemmas and strategies of theory construction. In: Snizek WE, Fuhrman ER, Miller MK, eds. *Contemporary Issues in Theory and Research: A Metasociological Perspective.* Westport, Conn: Greenwood Press; 1979.

Bova C. Adjustment to chronic illness among HIV-infected women. *J Nurs Sch.* 2001;33:217-223.

Carlson-Catalano J, Lunney M, Paradiso C, Bruno J, Luise BK, Martin T, et al. Clinical validation of ineffective breathing pattern, ineffective airway clearance, and impaired gas exchange. *Image.* 1998;30(3):243-248.

Coward DD. Critical multiplism: a research strategy for nursing science. *Image.* 1990;22:163-167.

Demerouti E, Bakker AB, Nachreiner F, Schaufeli WB. A model of burnout and life satisfaction amongst nurses. *J Adv Nurs.* 2000;32:454-464.

Doran DI, Sidani S, Keatings M, Doidge D. An empirical test of the Nursing Role Effectiveness Model. *J Adv Nurs.* 2002;38:29-39.

Ehrenberger HE, Alligood MR, Thomas SP, Wallace DC, Licavoli CM. Testing a theory of decision-making derived from King's systems framework in women eligible for a cancer clinical trial. *Nurs Sci Q.* 2002;15:156-163.

Fawcett J. *The Relationship of Theory and Research.* 3rd ed. Philadelphia, Penn: Davis; 1999.

Fehring R. Validating diagnostic labels: standardized methodology. In: Hurley ME, ed. *Classification of Nursing Diagnoses: Proceedings of the Sixth Conference.* St. Louis, Mo: Mosby; 1986.

Fiske DW, Shweder RA, eds. *Metatheory in Social Science.* Chicago, Ill: University of Chicago Press; 1986.

Frey MA, Rooke L, Sieloff C, Messmer PR, Kameoka T. King's framework and theory in Japan, Sweden, and the United States. *Image.* 1995;27:127-130.

Fry A, Nguyen T. Culture and the self: implications for the perception of depression by Australian and Vietnamese nursing students. *J Adv Nurs.* 1996;23:1147-1154.

Gordon M, Sweeney MA. Methodological problems and issues in identifying and standardizing nursing diagnoses. *Adv Nurs Sci.* 1979;2(1):1-15.

Hempel CG. *Philosophy of Natural Science.* Englewood Cliffs, NJ: Prentice Hall; 1966.

Hill PD, Humenick SS. Insufficient milk supply. *Image.* 1989;21:145-148.

Holter IM. Critical theory: a foundation for the development of nursing theories. *Scholar Inquiry Nurs Pract.* 1988;2:223-232.

Jennings-Dozier K. Predicting intentions to obtain a Pap smear among African American and Latina women: testing the theory of planned behavior. *Nurs Res.* 1999;48:198-205.

Johnson JL, Ratner PA, Bottorff JL, Hayduk LA. An exploration of Pender's health promotion model using Lisrel. *Nurs Res.* 1993;42:132-138.

Klaus MH, Jerauld R, Kreger MC, McAlpine W, Steffa M, Kennell JH. Maternal attachment: importance of the first postpartum days. *N Engl J Med.* 1972;286:460-463.

Klaus MH, Kennell JH. *Maternal–Infant Bonding.* St. Louis, Mo: Mosby; 1976.

Klaus MH, Kennell JH. *Parent–Infant Bonding.* 2nd ed. St. Louis, Mo: Mosby; 1982.

Marx MH. The general nature of theory construction. In: Marx MH, ed. *Theories in Contemporary Psychology.* New York, NY: Macmillan; 1963.

McCall RB. The media, society, and child development research. In: Osofsky JD, ed. *Handbook of Infant Development.* New York, NY: Wiley; 1987.

McCarley C. A model of chronic dyspnea. *Image.* 1999;31:231-236.

McCloskey JC, Bulechek GM. *Nursing Intervention Classification (NIC).* 3rd ed. St. Louis, Mo: Mosby; 2000.

McCullagh M, Lusk SL, Ronis DL. Factors influencing use of hearing protection among farmers: a test of the Pender Health Promotion Model. *Nurs Res.* 2002;51:33-39.

Nagley SJ, Byers PH. Clinical construct validity. *J Adv Nurs.* 1987;12:617-619.

Nivens AS, Herman J, Weinrich SP, Weinrich MC. Cues to participation in prostate cancer screening: a theory for practice. *Oncol Nurs Forum.* 2001;28:1449-1156.

Pedhazur EJ, Schmelkin LP. *Measurement, Design, and Analysis: An Integrated Approach.* Hillsdale, NJ: Erlbaum; 1991.

Pender NJ. *Health Promotion in Nursing Practice.* 2nd ed. Norwalk, Conn: Appleton & Lange; 1987.

Phillips DC. *Philosophy, Science, and Social Inquiry.* New York, NY: Pergamon Press; 1987.

Platt JR. Strong inference. *Science.* 1964;146:347-352.

Polit DF, Beck CT. *Nursing Research: Principles and Methods.* 7th ed. Philadelphia, Penn: Lippincott; 2003.

Popper KR. *Conjectures and Refutations.* New York, NY: Basic Books; 1965.

Potempa K, Lopez M, Reid C, Lawson L. Chronic fatigue. *Image.* 1986;18:165-169.

Schumacher KL, Gortner SR. (Mis)conceptions and reconceptions about traditional science. *Adv Nurs Sci.* 1992;14(4):1-11.

Silva MC. Research testing nursing theory: state of the art. *Adv Nurs Sci.* 1986;9(1):1-11.

Silva MC, Sorrell JM. Testing of nursing theory: critique and philosophical expansion. *Adv Nurs Sci.* 1992;14(4):12-23.

Susser M. Maternal weight gain, infant birth weight, and diet: causal sequences. *Am J Clin Nutr.* 1991;53:1384-1396.

Tabachnick BG, Fidell LS. *Using Multivarite Statistics.* 4th ed. Boston, Mass: Pearson, Allen & Bacon; 2001.

Villarruel AM. Mexican-American cultural meanings, expressions, self-care and dependent-care actions associated with experiences of pain. *Res Nurs Health.* 1995;18:427-436.

Villarruel AM, Denyes MJ. Testing Orem's theory with Mexican Americans. *Image.* 1997;29:283-288.

Wallace WL. *The Logic of Science in Sociology.* New York, NY: Aldine; 1971.

Waltz CF, Strickland OL, Lenz ER. *Measurement in Nursing Research.* 2nd ed. Philadelphia, Penn: Davis; 1991.

Yeh C. Health-related quality of life in pediatric patients with cancer: a structural equation approach with the Roy Adaptation Model. *Cancer Nurs.* 2002;25:74-80.

Zauszniewski JA, Chung C, Krafcik K. Social cognitive factors predicting the health of elders. *West J Nurs Res.* 2001;23:490-503.

ADDITIONAL READINGS

Acton GJ, Irvin BL, Hopkins BA. Theory-testing research: building the science. *Adv Nurs Sci.* 1991;14(1):52-61.

Behi R, Nolan M. Deduction: moving from the general to the specific. *Br J Nurs.* 1995;4:341-344.

Coates VE. Measuring constructs accurately: a prerequisite to theory testing. *J Psychiatr Ment Health Nurs.* 1995;2:287-293.

Dulock HL, Holzemer WL. Substruction: improving the linkage from theory to research. *Nurs Sci Q.* 1991;4:83-87.

Fawcett J. Testing nursing theory. In: *Analysis and Evaluation of Nursing Theories.* Philadelphia, Penn: Lippincott; 1993.

Field M. Causal inference in behavioral research. *Adv Nurs Sci.* 1979;2(1):81-93.

Gibbs JP. Part 3: test of theories. In: *Sociological Theory Construction.* Hinsdale, Ill: Dryden Press; 1972.

Hall JM, Stevens PE. Rigor in feminist research. *Adv Nurs Sci.* 1991;13(3):16-29.

Hinshaw AS. Theoretical model testing: full utilization of data. *West J Nurs Res.* 1984;6:5-9.

Jacobs MK. Can nursing theory be tested? In: Chinn PL, ed. *Nursing Research Methodology.* Rockville, Md: Aspen; 1986.

McQuiston CM, Campbell JC. Theoretical substruction: a guide for theory testing research. *Nurs Sci Q.* 1997;10:117-123.

Mullins NC. Empirical testing. In: *The Art of Theory: Construction and Use.* New York, NY: Harper & Row; 1971.

Reynolds PD. Testing theories. In: *A Primer in Theory Construction.* Indianapolis, Ind: Bobbs-Merrill; 1971.

Sandelowski M. The problem of rigor in qualitative research. *Adv Nurs Sci.* 1986;8(3):27-37.

Wallace WL. Tests of hypotheses; decisions to accept or reject hypotheses; logical inference; theories. In: *The Logic of Science of Sociology.* New York, NY: Aldine; 1971.

Zetterberg HL. *On Theory and Verification in Sociology.* Totowa, NJ: Bedminster Press; 1965.

13

Frontiers of Nursing Theory and Knowledge Development

Preliminary Note: *Predicting the future is risky business at best. Although we cannot know what trends will predominate within nursing theory development in the future, we can identify areas that appear to be vigorously expanding. Our consideration of the areas we chose to focus on below reflect both the growing breadth as well as the increasing depth of nursing theory and knowledge development.*

INTRODUCTION

In this final chapter we focus on two frontiers of nursing knowledge that emerged in our review of the literature for this fourth edition: (1) progress in international and ethnicity-related nursing theory, and (2) the tandem areas of nursing informatics and evidence-based practice. Our treatment is necessarily selective in nature and limited to English-language sources.

ADVANCES IN INTERNATIONAL AND ETHNICITY-RELATED NURSING THEORY

Probably the most tangible landmarks documenting the growth of international and ethnicity-related nursing theory and knowledge development are the presence of nursing journals, such as the *Journal of Advanced Nursing* from the United Kingdom, *Theoria, Journal of Nursing Theory* from Sweden (Willman, 2000), and the *Journal of National Black Nurses Association* from the United States. Two U.S. journals also are noteworthy in their fostering of international scholarship related to nursing theory or knowledge development: *Nursing Science Quarterly* and *Journal of Nursing Scholarship* (formerly *Image*).These and other journals like them serve several purposes. They give concrete evidence of the growing numbers of scholars concerned with the needs of specific international and ethnic populations. They provide nurses with an added outlet for disseminating their theory and research related to populations of interest. They bring to nurses who serve the populations of interest the latest advances in theory and related research. More broadly, the growth in international nursing knowledge development is supported by a survey published in *Journal of Nursing Scholarship* summarizing international publishing outlets in English-language nursing journals from 13 countries (McConnell, 2000). Thus, we draw on some of these as well as other sources for our review below.

International Nursing Theory Development

Addressing the international literature on nursing theory is fraught with difficulties because theoretical thinking often grows in an interactional context so that it is not always fully reflected in published literature. Searches of literature databases may uncover articles of interest in non-English-language journals, but costs imposed by the need for translation may make those sources beyond easy reach. Bearing in mind these challenges, we judged the topic of international work in nursing theory development to be important enough to warrant the risks involved. For feasibility, we focused on articles published in English. Our coverage, thus, is only a partial consideration of international efforts at nursing theory development. Furthermore, because of the breadth of international theory development literature, our review is necessarily selective and illustrative. (Also see Additional Readings at the end of this chapter.)

To begin, among the controversies conveyed in theory-related articles by international authors were statements for the value and contribution of theory (Allison, McLaughlin, & Walker, 1991; Biley & Biley, 2001; Draper, 1990; Poggenpoel, 1996; Searle, 1988); concern about the uncritical adoption of U.S.-based nursing theories, values, and knowledge schemes (Draper, 1990; Ketefian & Redman, 1997; Lawler, 1991); questioning the need for unique nursing knowledge (Nolan, Lundh, & Tishelman, 1998); disparagement or questioning of grand theories (Daly & Jackson, 1999; Nolan et al., 1998); advocating contextual or delimited scope theories (Daly & Jackson, 1999; Draper, 1990; Nolan et al., 1998); and questioning the effectiveness of imposing theories using a top-down strategy (Kenney, 1993). For example, Nolan et al. (1998) argued that grand nursing theories fail to meet the needs of practice because they are too far removed from reality to be useful to practitioners.

These controversies indicate a growing awareness that it is important to understand that theoretical work based on the American experience may need to be modified to fit other countries, or may be incompatible with cultural and other considerations for application in some countries. Nonetheless, where cross-national and global knowledge-related efforts are reasonable to pursue, they offer the opportunity for more widespread benefit and enhanced progress on theoretical and knowledge-related outcomes. Such efforts also offer potential for collaborative work that ideally benefits all partners. Because of migration and international travel, knowledge that can "cross borders" prevents the age-old problem of "reinventing the wheel." Nursing diagnosis and related nomenclature has been one such area of international collaboration (Casey, 2002; Ehnfors, 2002; Goosen, 2002; Ketefian & Redman, 1997). However, the expansion of nursing diagnoses and related systems of classification are not without their detractors (Lawler, 1991; Nolan et al., 1998).

TABLE 13–1   EXAMPLES OF INTERNATIONAL DISCOURSE ON NURSING THEORY

Author Country or Countries	Author(s)	Topic or Focus
Australia	Emden & Young, 1987	Integrative review of "trends and issues" in nursing theory development; Delphi study
Sweden and Norway	Lundh, Söder, & Waerness, 1988	Critique of nursing process and nursing theories
United Kingdom	Draper, 1990	Contributions of nursing theory and impediments to its development in the United Kingdom
Australia	Holden, 1991	Critical examination of dualism, idealism, and materialism as theories of mind applied in nursing
United Kingdom	Reed & Robbins, 1991	Proposed and illustrated inductive theory "testing"
Australia	Bruni, 1991	Discourse analysis of literature related to nursing as a profession and knowledge development
Sweden	Dahlberg, 1994	Exposition of holistic perspective and gender-related barriers to application in practice
Sweden	Lutzen & da Silva, 1995	Linguistic issues, nursing methodology, concept of care, trends
Australia	Holmes, 1996	Summary of postmodern critiques of traditional science; alternative philosophic stances for nursing summarized
Canada	Baker, 1997	Critical analysis of cultural relativism, including its use in nursing theories
United Kingdom and Sweden	Nolan, Lundh, & Tishelman, 1998	Critique grand nursing theory, critique unique nursing knowledge, advocate middle-range theory
Korea	Shin, 2001	Taoism, Buddhism, and Confucianism as related to nursing theory in Korea

A number of nurses have reported on the conceptual, metatheoretical, historical, or educational issues and achievements related to developing and applying nursing theory within specific countries, such as the following: Sweden (Lutzen & da Silva, 1995; Willman & Stoltz, 2002), United Kingdom (Smith, 1987), Canada (Major, Pepin, & Légault, 2001; Rodgers, 2000), Australia (Daly & Jackson, 1999), Finland (Leino-Kilpi & Suominen, 1998), Japan (Hisama, 2001), Iceland (Jonsdottir, 2001), India (Sirra, 1986), and South Africa (Searle, 1988). Furthermore, an array of metatheoretical and philosophical topics are addressed in the international literature related to nursing theory; illustrative examples are displayed in Table 13–1. In a contribution unique in the international literature, Emden and Young (1987) reported on a Delphi study conducted with nursing experts on issues related to theory development in Australia. Expert opinion was sought on seven issues, such as whether nursing theory development was "critical to the advancement of professional nursing" and "nursing should develop its own unique research traditions" (p. 27). Detailed presentation of the expert opinions on issue statements represents one of the few studies of this kind and would, no doubt, be of interest to readers in a number of countries outside Australia.

International literature on theory development also embraces theorizing about abstract representations of nursing and nursing values, such as, the Roper-Logan-Tierney (1985) nursing model; Andersen's (1991) nursing activity model; Eriksson's (2002) exposition of caring science; Sarvimäki's (1988) theory of nursing care; Chao's concept of caring (1992); and Minshull, Ross, and Turner's (1986) human needs nursing model. Other theoretical efforts have focused on critiquing and applying nursing theories. For example, Tierney (1998) examined the contributions and criticisms of the Roper-Logan-Tierney (1985) nursing model. Whall, Shin, and Colling (1999) examined a derivative of Nightingale's thought for suitability to care of cognitively impaired elders in Korea, whereas Clift and Barrett (1998) tested a power framework in three German-speaking countries, and da Nobrega and Coler (1994) used nursing theory as a basis of nursing diagnoses in Brazil. Examples of still other works include explicating nurses' practice models for patients with dermatological conditions (Lauri, Salanterä, Chalmers, Ekman, Kim, Käppeli, et al., 2001), decision making in adult and gerontology care settings (Kirkevold, 1993), analysis of a pediatric care model (Lee, 1998), and development or application of theory to the care of psychiatric patients (Mavundla, Poggenpoel, & Gmeiner, 2001; Poggenpoel, 1996).

Theories of U.S. origin have also been the subject of application internationally as well as critique. For example, de Villiers and van der Wal (1995) applied Leininger's (1991) model to curriculum development in South Africa, whereas Bruni (1988) critiqued earlier elements of the theory. Similarly Morales-Mann and Jiang (1993) critically examined Orem's (1991) theory in the light of fit with Chinese culture, whereas Lauder (2001) critiqued it in relation to self-neglect. In a related vein, Baker (1997) critically examined the issue of cultural relativism in nursing theory and practice. Examples of still other U.S.-origin nursing theories applied internationally include a multinational study using Parse's (1999) theory (Baumann, 2002), and application and testing of King's (1981) theory within three countries (Frey, Rooke, Sieloff, Messmer, & Kameoka, 1995). No doubt there are many other examples of theory applications that we are overlooking.

In conclusion, the international literature related to nursing theory that we reviewed is rich and diverse, despite being limited to English-language sources. The range of theoretical works includes metatheoretical and critical work, and covers a variety of needs and contexts. There is no evidence of one predominating theory in the literature that we reviewed. Indeed, there was much skepticism about imposing theories from outside a country. We expect to see an exponential increase in international literature related to nursing theory in the future.

Ethnicity-Related Nursing Theory Development

Because of the cultural, racial, and ethnic diversity of the United States, our consideration of ethnicity-related knowledge and theory development will be directed primarily at certain theoretical advances in the U.S. context, but may be applica-

ble to similarly diverse countries. As with international nursing theory, our literature review is limited to sources that we discovered primarily through hand
searches. The minimal number of sources found through computerized searches
may indicate a limitation of descriptors attached to nursing theory-related articles
pertaining to ethnic populations. Omission of a work in our review may simply reflect the limits of our search methods and is not a statement of a work's importance.

As in the international literature, a key concern expressed within literature focused on ethnic minority populations was potential mismatch between the views
and values inherent in extant nursing theories and those held by ethnic minority
populations. Orem's (1991) theory was an example of a grand theory analyzed for
such potential incongruence. For example, Roberson and Kelley (1996) proposed
that Orem's theory reflects Western values such as self-reliance and self-direction
that may be incongruent in cultural groups that value interdependence and har-
mony. They further propose that the biomedical orientation in Orem's theory may
be incongruent with folk health practices. In a review of several international and
U.S.-based studies, Roberson and Kelley concluded that the theory insufficiently
delineated how culture affects health, thereby limiting "the theory's usefulness for
guiding culturally competent nursing care" (p. 27). In an analysis of an inductive
study couched in Orem's (1991) theory, Villarruel and Denyes (1997) reported
that self-care agency and dependent-care agency (separate terms in Orem's theory)
were difficult to differentiate in their study of Mexican Americans. They noted that
caring for others was highly valued among participants from this cultural group.

Because of concern about the misfit of theories developed from a dominant culture perspective when applied to ethnic minority groups, efforts have been undertaken to develop frameworks, concepts, and perspectives that reflect specific cultural
groups. At the concept level, Dancy and colleagues (2001) explored the concept of
empowerment within two African American urban housing projects. After reviewing the literature on empowerment, they documented the impact of the urban housing project environments on the outreach team members' observations, feelings, and
thoughts. Using content analysis, they explored the negative impact of the housing
project environment on their own feelings of empowerment. Im and Meleis (1999)
applied the idea of situation-specific theory to investigate the phenomenon of
menopause among Korean immigrants to the United States. Their findings derived
from this specific group of women were then used to modify a more general model
of transition experiences. Loxe and Struthers (2001) used focus group data to design
a nursing conceptual framework for Native American culture. Examples of key concepts in the conceptual framework were the following: caring, traditions, respect,
and holism. In a related work, Jensen-Wunder (2002) developed a nursing practice
model from her experiences with a Lakota community. Starting from a commitment
to human becoming (Parse, 1995), Jensen-Wunder developed the model, Indian
Health Initiatives, using symbols and beliefs derived from Lakota culture.

Critical scholarship methods and ways of knowing have been applied to ar-
ticulation of frameworks and methodologies for study of cultural groups and
cultural-gender groups. Turton (1997), for example, developed the health-world

view orienting framework for ethnographic research on health promotion among the Ojibwe community. Boutain (1999) proposed combining critical social theory and African American studies methods as a more powerful way for nurses to study the health and social context of African Americans. Two other nurses described womanism (Taylor, 1998) and womanist ways of knowing (Banks-Wallace, 2000) as forms of gender-centered thought of value to nursing scholarship focused on the context and health of African American women.

In conclusion, important beginning contributions are being made for developing nursing theory that is congruent with the cultural context of ethnic minority populations in the United States. Given the U.S. demographic changes, concern for the health of ethnic minority populations, and efforts to eliminate health disparities faced by them, further development of theory in nursing in this area is an important priority.

NURSING INFORMATICS AND EVIDENCE-BASED PRACTICE

Although the fields of informatics and evidence-based practice seem relatively "new" in the last two decades, the issues of good documentation, adequate information to inform decisions, and best practices have been around since formal nursing began. It seems informatics and evidence-based practices have been uniquely interrelated phenomena of concern to nurses throughout our history.

> *In attempting to arrive at the truth, I have applied everywhere for information, but in scarcely an instance have I been able to obtain hospital records fit for any purpose of comparison. If they could be obtained they would enable us to decide many other questions besides the one alluded to. They would show the subscribers how their money was being spent, what good was really being done with it, or whether the money was not doing mischief rather than good; . . . And if wisely used, these improved statistics would tell more the relative value of particular operations and modes of treatment than we have means of ascertaining at present. They would enable us, besides, to ascertain the influence of the hospital . . . upon the course of operations and diseases passing through its wards; and the truth thus ascertained would enable us to save life and suffering and to improve the treatment and management of the sick. (Nightingale, 1863, pp. 175–176)*

Miss Nightingale had it right 150 years ago. There is a significant link between good evidence and the outcomes of nursing work. Nurses rely heavily on sufficient, appropriate, and timely information in the delivery of care. Without sufficient and appropriate information, decision making is hampered and quality of care is jeopardized. The quality and types of information available significantly impact upon the kinds and quality of decisions made. As Miss Nightingale suggested, whether needed information is *available and retrievable* for use also impacts on quality of patient outcomes and decisions made. In fact, Ireson and Velotta (1998) suggest that seeming unwillingness to *use* evidence in practice is, in part, due to nurses being unable to retrieve evidence or needing evidence that is not available. This problem accounts for the often 10-year lag-time between completion of research studies and use of the findings in practice.

Nurses don't just use information; they *produce* it as well, and on a daily basis. Whether it is documenting in a patient record, writing clinical guidelines, or publishing research findings, nurses are expected to provide evidence of their practice. The quality of the information they produce and how that information is stored and maintained also significantly affects how it is used. Without adequate production of information and evidence, nursing care and decisions are also hampered (Bakken-Henry, 1995).

Definitions of Evidence-Based Practice and Informatics

Definitions of the two fields demonstrate their interconnectedness. **Evidence-based practice (EBP)** has been defined in several ways. Sackett et al. (1996) define it as "the conscientious, explicit and judicious use of current best evidence about the care of individual patients . . . integrating individual clinical expertise with the best available external clinical evidence from systematic research" (p. 71). French (2002) refers to it as "the systematic interconnecting of scientifically generated evidence with the tacit knowledge of the expert practitioner to achieve a change in a particular practice for the benefit of a well defined client/patient group" (p. 74). Roberts (1998) states, "EBP uses evidence gleaned from research to establish sound clinical practice" (p. 24). Finally, Eisenberg (1998) contends that "evidence-based clinical practice draws on the findings of research to provide information to improve patient care for each individual, while at the same time challenging researchers to address the questions for which clinicians and patients most urgently need information." Of course, a theorist must *have* evidence before he or she has evidence-based practice. Decisions that are evidence based are often hampered because many interventions have limited formal research evidence to support them (Millenson, 1997). The situation is improving, but lack of sufficient evidence impedes the implementation of evidence-based practice.

Nursing informatics has been defined as "a combination of computer science, information science and nursing science designed to assist in the management and processing of nursing data, information and knowledge to support the practice of nursing and the delivery of nursing care" (Graves & Corcoran, 1989, p. 227). Hannah, Ball, & Edwards (1994) define it as "the use of information technologies in relation to those functions within the purview of nursing, and that are carried out by nurses when performing their duties" (p. 3). Finally, Turley (1996) calls nursing informatics "the interaction of cognitive science, computer science, and information science resting on a base of nursing science" (p. 309). Informatics provides some of the infrastructure for managing, storing, retrieving, and working with various forms of nursing data, information, and evidence.

Heller, Oros, and Durney-Crowley (2000) cite 10 trends that they believe will be highly significant factors in nursing in the 21st century. Three of the trends are highly relevant to this discussion. First is the technological explosion, which enumerates the dramatic changes in computers, information systems, and telecommunications; technologic changes in patient care and diagnostics; and improvements in accessibility of clinical data. A second trend relates to the cost of health care, the changes in health care systems, and the lack of insurance coverage by huge numbers of persons. A third trend, the significant advance in nursing science and research, highlights the increasing numbers of studies that provide a scientific basis for nursing care to improve patient outcomes. Thus, 3 of the 10 trends related directly to informatics and evidence-based practice, emphasizing the importance these two trends will have over the next few years.

Although there is some concern about the current emphasis on evidence-based practice for nursing (French, 2002; Jennings, 2000; Jennings & Loan, 2001) because it is philosophically based on the medical evidence-based model (EBM), we believe that evidence of good practice is always important. However, the concerns are also valid ones that need to be kept in mind during any discussion of evidence-based practice in particular. The concerns are expressed because the medical EBM focuses *only* on medical diagnosis, single interventions, and meta-analyses, and uses the gold standard for evidence as the randomized controlled trial (RCT; Kitson, 1997). Jennings and French both point out that nurses have misunderstood the term and its underlying intent and question whether nursing really wants to concentrate large portions of energy *only* on specific interventions and RCTs. Nurses who espouse using evidence-based practice because they think it will help them achieve better quality care across the spectrum of nursing arenas and help them demonstrate "how nursing works," may want to be very specific about what they mean when they use the term. The potential for nursing scientists to be misled by using a term that is not fully comprehended may catapult nursing science into a situation where it is severely constrained in its purposes and scope. For the purpose of this book we prefer to use the broader understanding of evidence-based practice that includes any of the following: any steps in the nursing process (assessment, diagnosis, goal setting, interventions, outcomes, or evaluation), decision support, quality improvements, standards and guidelines, and workload evaluations and staffing.

Growth of the Ideas

Although the issue of evidence for use in practice and decision support has been around since Nightingale, the advent of inexpensive and very efficient computers and information systems has pushed health care systems and health care workers into the information age with a vengeance. The amazing growth of electronic patient records has significantly changed the way patient care is documented. In addition, there has been a relative explosion of nursing research related to interventions, outcomes, effectiveness of care, cost of care, and so forth.

As a result, there has been a remarkable increase in nursing informatics activities in the last several years. Several universities now have majors in nursing informatics at master's and doctoral levels. In addition there are journals devoted exclusively to nursing informatics, such as *Computers in Nursing, Online Journal of Nursing Informatics,* and *CIN: Computers, Informatics, Nursing,* and a host of books. There are also journals that publish nursing informatics articles but are not exclusively nursing focused—for instance, *Journal of the American Informatics Association* and *Topics in Health Information Management.* There is even certification available as an informatics nurse. There are nursing informatics professional organizations (American Nursing Informatics Association, Nursing Informatics Special Interest Group of the International Medical Informatics Association, American Health Information Management Association, and the Ontario Informatics Group to name but a few). Informatics conferences are held all over the world.

Likewise, there has been a significant increase in the emphasis on evidence-based practice as demonstrated by an increasing number of books (e.g., Martin, Rodrigues, Delaney, Nielsen, & Yan, 2001; Moorhead & Delaney, 1998) and articles in nursing journals (French, 2002) in addition to the publication of at least one specialized nursing journal (*Evidence-Based Nursing*), published by the Royal College of Nursing in Great Britain. There are even specialized libraries, such as the Cochrane Library, available where evidence-based care research is housed.

We found definite clusters of articles in the literature we reviewed. Table 13–2 lists the major categories and the authors of the articles we reviewed. The full citations can be found in the References at the end of the chapter. It is beyond the scope of this chapter to abstract each article. However, issues raised in several of these are discussed in the next section.

Model and Theory Development in Informatics and Evidence-Based Practice

Most of the theoretical work was in the evidence-based practice domain. Very little was found in the informatics literature in nursing with the exception of Turley's (1996) model discussed later. This is not to say that informatics lacks a theoretical base, but it does tend to be information science based; it is not focused on nursing theory.

However, in five articles the authors called for better theoretical underpinnings for evidence-based practice and decision making and the knowledge development that drives these efforts (Elkan, Blair, & Robinson, 2000; Fawcett, Watson, Neuman, Walker, & Fitzpatrick, 2001; Liehr & Smith, 1999; Thompson, 1999; Walker, 1999). Although each took a somewhat different approach, each suggested that integrating and expanding what nursing views as evidence would promote growth of knowledge and allow for sound middle-range theory development in nursing. Each suggested that evidence-based practice and the research that directs it should be theory based. This approach would allow for a more comprehensive view of nursing knowledge as it guides practice. Three of the articles actually proposed models or methods for theory development (Elkan et al., Fawcett et al., and Thompson). This is encouraging to see. For the first several years of the movement toward evidence-based practice, there was little mention of theory as a basis for evidence, or vice versa.

Taking a slightly different approach, Blegen and Tripp-Reimer (1997) suggest that established taxonomies of nursing languages might constitute the basis for middle-range theory development for nursing practice. They contend that linking nursing diagnosis concepts with interventions to predict expected outcomes is a reasonable way to construct theory that is relevant to and supports evidence-based practice.

Four articles reported meta-analyses on the effects of psychoeducational care in adults with asthma (Devine, 1996), the effects of a fall prevention program for elderly people (Hill-Westmoreland, Soeken, & Spellbring, 2002), and predictors

TABLE 13–2 SUMMARY OF SELECTED LITERATURE RELATED TO EVIDENCE-BASED PRACTICE AND INFORMATICS

Categories of Articles	Authors and Dates
Effectiveness of nursing	American Hospital Association Commission of Workforce, 2002 Kimball & O'Neil, 2001 Mason, 1999 Needleman, Buerhaus, Mattke, Stewart, & Zelevinsky, 2002 Wong et al., 2002
Decision support and expert systems	Effken, 2001 Facione & Facione, 1996 Greenwood, Sullivan, Spence, & McDonald, 2000 Hallett, Austin, Caress, & Luker, 2000 Harding, Redmond, Corley, & Nelson, 1996 Laschinger, Sabiston, & Kutszcher, 1997 Narayan & Corcoran-Perry, 1997 Radwin, 1995
Standardized language development	Aquilino, 1997 Bjornsdottir, 2001 Bliss-Holtz, 1996 Bowles & Naylor, 1996 Broome, 1999 Coenan, Marek, & Lundeen, 1996 Foster, 2001 Frisch, 1997 Iowa Intervention Project, 1997 Lavin, Meyer, & Carlson, 1999 Maas, Johnson, & Moorhead, 1996 Moorhead & Delaney, 1997 Simon, 1998 Snyder, Egan, & Nojima, 1996 Wake & Coenan, 1998 Whitely, 1999 Zielstorff, Tronni, Basque, Griffin, & Welebob, 1998
Quality of care and quality improvement	Clark, 2000 Leveck & Jones, 1996 Prowse & Lyne, 2000 Thomas, Cullum, & McColl, 1998 Thomas, McColl, & Cullum, 1998
Integrating research and practice	Gamel, Grypdonck, Hengeveld, & Davis, 2001 Jairath & Fain, 1999 McCormack, Kitson, Harvey, Rycroft-Malone, Titchen, & Seers, 2002
Technology development and use	Alexander & Kroposki, 2001 Alpay & Russell, 2002 Barnard, 2000 Gurrieri, 2000 Keenan et al., 2002 Nicoll, 2001 Norris, 1999 Sparks & Rizzolo, 1998 Timmons, 2002

of postpartum depression (Beck, 1996a, 1996b). Although each looked at the effectiveness of either predictors or interventions, none proposed a theory or a model of the findings. Such meta-analyses are considered in the EBM hierarchy as very strong evidence for practice. The authors made careful recommendations about potentials for practice. However, these recommendations did not consider how the strength of the evidence related to the potential for theory development.

Three articles proposed development of middle-range theory based on the use of clinical guidelines (Gooch, 1991; Good & Moore, 1996) and standards of care (Ruland & Moore, 1998). The authors suggest that guidelines and standards are fruitful grounds for developing middle-range theory that is directly linked to practice. They argue that standards and guidelines directly link to nursing interventions and outcomes. Good and Moore even propose a method for developing theory from guidelines and demonstrate how it can be done. The result leads to a theory synthesis (see Chapter 9) that is relevant to practice.

In a somewhat related article, Traynor, Rafferty, and Lewison (2001) conducted a bibliometric study of all biomedical research in the United Kingdom. (Bibliometrics is the study of citation patterns in the literature.) They found that nursing research was the fourth-ranking category of publications in their analysis. Nursing topics ranged widely across the discipline. They also suggested that using meta-analysis was a good basis for establishing guidelines for evidence-based practice.

Three articles actually proposed models or theories related to evidence-based practice or informatics. Kolcaba (2001) presented a fascinating discussion of the development of the mid-range theory of comfort and its eventual use for outcomes research. She carefully detailed the steps taken to build and refine the theory and demonstrated how using the theory in outcomes research not only benefited the patients, but also some institutional outcomes related to nurse productivity. Smith and colleagues (2002) used the caregiving effectiveness model to predict the outcomes of family members' caregiving on technology-dependent elders in the home. The authors found that nurses were very willing to use the verified relational statements in the model to generate nursing interventions. Mitchell, Ferketich, Jennings, and the American Academy of Nursing Expert Panel on Quality Health Care (1998) proposed a dynamic model for quality health outcomes. They suggested that the model is broad enough to allow for research on system level interventions and outcomes at both individual and systems levels, to guide formation of relevant clinical databases, and to help researchers identify key variables for study. It is extremely encouraging to see this beginning interest in the theoretical underpinnings of evidence-based practice. We hope that a similar upsurge of interest in nursing informatics theory will emerge within the next few years.

The only theory proposed for informatics in the literature we reviewed was that by Turley (1996). Turley proposed that nursing informatics be based within the three fields of cognitive science, computer science, and information science, but resting on a base of nursing science. He envisioned a model of three-dimensional Venn diagrams encapsulated within the science base of nursing. He proposed that research is needed at each of the intersections within the model, but all of it be focused within the context of nursing. Certainly, we look forward to seeing what may come from the use of this model. It provides a very clear view of the field of nursing informatics.

SOME FINAL MUSINGS

We have been very impressed with the amount of theoretical work done to date relating to nursing theory and knowledge development. We hope that such strides in development will continue over the course of the next several years. With the large numbers of young researchers entering the ranks, we look forward to exciting new theory development across the globe. We continue to urge novice researchers and theorists to "think outside the box," be fearless in trying new ideas, and most of all, enjoy the process.

Information technology now drives much of our communications, keeps us in touch with each other and the world, and provides consumers with instant information about health care services, new drugs, and the latest in health technology. Consumers are becoming very knowledgeable about best practices related to their particular health situations. It is important that nurses keep up to date with the rapid development of such technology and to use it appropriately.

Although evidence may vary by type and source, as we have said earlier, one of the first criteria for evidence is that it be available and retrievable so it can be used. Developing theories related to informatics use in practice can provide direction to programmers, software developers, and vendors. Such theories may assist in determining what nursing data are relevant to input, store, maintain, and retrieve, and how to represent that data in their products. Without adequate theories of what nursing information is critical and how the data types are related to each other, developers and vendors cannot be responsive to nursing's particular needs for evidence to advance practice.

Finally, our review of evidenced-based practice brings us full circle to issues presented in Chapter 1 related to the historical context of nursing knowledge development. The idea that nursing practice is evidence based represents the fulfillment of the earlier ideas of Bixler and Bixler (1945) wherein "a well-defined and well-organized body of specialized knowledge" (p. 730) was proposed as a requirement of professional status of nursing. For nursing, however, practice must be not only evidence based but also theory based. In other words, in nursing, values and perspectives of the patient or client are central to the care process. Those values and perspectives, though often criticized as overly "grand," remain the benchmarks for what gives nursing its distinctive view of care among the health professions.

REFERENCES

Alexander JW, Kroposki, M. Using a management perspective to define and measure changes in nursing technology. *J Adv Nurs.* 2001;35(5):776-778.

Allison SE, McLaughlin K, Walker D. Nursing theory: a tool to put nursing back into nursing administration. *Nurs Adm Q.* 1991;15(3):72-78.

Alpay L, Russell A. Information technology training in primary care: the nurses' voice. *CIN: Computers, Informatics, Nursing.* 2002;20(4):136-142.

Andersen BM. Mapping the terrain of the discipline. In: Gray G, Pratt R, eds. *Towards a Discipline of Nursing.* Melbourne, Australia: Churchill Livingstone; 1991.

Aquilino ML. Cognitive development, clinical knowledge, and clinical experience related to diagnostic ability. *Nurs Diagn.* 1997;8(3):110-118.

Baker C. Cultural relativism and cultural diversity: implications for nursing practice. *Adv Nurs Sci.* 1997;20(1):3-11.

Bakken-Henry S. Informatics: essential infrastructure for quality assessment and improvement in nursing. *J Amer Med Informatics Assoc.* 1995;2:169-182.

Banks-Wallace J. Womanist ways of knowing: theoretical considerations for research with African American women. *Adv Nurs Sci.* 2000;22(3):33-45.

Barnard A. Alteration in will as an experience of technology and nursing. *J Adv Nurs.* 2000;31(5):1136-1145.

Baumann SL. Toward a global perspective of the human sciences. *Nurs Sci Q.* 2002;15:381-384.

Beck CT. A meta-analysis of predictors of postpartum depression. *Nurs Res.* 1996a;45(5):297-303.

Beck CT. A meta-analysis of the relationship between postpartum depression and infant temperament. *Nurs Res.* 1996b;45(4):225-230.

Biley A, Biley FC. Nursing models and theories: more than just passing fads. *Theoria J Nurs Theory.* 2001;10(2):5-10.

Bixler G, Bixler RW. The professional status of nursing. *Amer J Nurs.* 1945;45:730-735.

Bjornsdottir K. Language, research and nursing practice. *J Adv Nurs.* 2001;33(2):159-166.

Blegen MA, Tripp-Reimer T. Implications of nursing taxonomies for middle-range theory development. *Adv Nurs Sci.* 1997;19(3):37-49.

Bliss-Holtz J. Using Orem's theory to generate nursing diagnoses for electronic documentation. *Nurs Sci Q.* 1996;9(3):121-125.

Boutain DM. Critical nursing scholarship: exploring critical social theory with African American studies. *Adv Nurs Sci.* 1999;21(4):37-47.

Bowles KH, Naylor MD. Nursing intervention classification systems. *Image.* 1996;28(4):303-308.

Broome ME. Outcomes research: practice counts! *J Soc Pediatr Nurses.* 1999;4(2):83-84.

Bruni N. A critical analysis of transcultural theory. *Aust J Adv Nurs.* 1988;5(3):26-32.

Bruni N. Nursing knowledge: processes of production. In: Gray G, Pratt R, eds. *Towards a Discipline of Nursing.* Melbourne, Australia: Churchill Livingstone; 1991.

Casey A. Standardization and nursing terminology. In: Oud N, ed. *ACENDIO 2002: Proceedings of the Special Conference of the Association of Common European Nursing Diagnoses, Interventions and Outcomes in Vienna.* Bern, Switzerland: Verlag Hans Huber; 2002.

Chao S. Review: nursing care driven by guidelines improves some process measures and patient outcomes. *Cochrane Rev.* 1991;2(3):87.

Chao Y. A unique concept of nursing care. *Int Nurs Rev.* 1992;39(6):181-184.

Clark J. Old wine in new bottles: delivering nursing in the 21st century. *J Nurs Sch.* 2000; 32(1):11-15.

Clift J, Barrett E. Testing nursing theory cross-culturally. *Int Nurs Rev.* 1998;45(4):123-126, 128.

Coenan A, Marek KD, Lundeen SP. Using nursing diagnoses to explain utilization in a community nursing center. *Res Nurs Health.* 1996;19:441-445.

Dahlberg K. The collision between caring theory and caring practice as a collision between feminine and masculine cognitive style. *J Holistic Nurs.* 1994;12:391-401.

Daly J, Jackson D. On the use of nursing theory in nurse education, nursing practice, and nursing research in Australia. *Nurs Sci Q.* 1999;12:342-345.

Dancy BL, McCreary L, Daye M, Wright J, Simpson S, Williams C. Empowerment: a view of two low-income African-American communities. *J Natl Black Nurses Assoc.* 2001;12:49-52.

da Nobrega MML, Coler MS. The utilization of Horta's Basic Human Needs Theory in the identification and classification of nursing diagnoses in Brazil. In: Carroll-Johnson RM, Paquette M, eds. *Classification of Nursing Diagnoses: Proceedings of the Tenth Conference.* Philadelphia, Penn: Lippincott; 1994.

de Villiers L, van der Wal D. Putting Leininger's nursing theory "culture care diversity and universality" into operation in the curriculum—part 1. *Curationis.* 1995;18(4):56-60.

Devine EC. Meta-analysis of the effects of psychoeducational care in adults with asthma. *Res Nurs Health.* 1996;19:367-376.

diCenso A, Cullum N, Ciliska D, eds. *Evidence-Based Nursing Journal.* Vol 1-7. London, England: Royal College of Nursing; 1998–2004.

Draper P. The development of theory in British nursing: current position and future prospects. *J Adv Nurs.* 1990;15(1):12-15.

Effken JA. Informational basis for expert intuition. *J Adv Nurs.* 2001;34(2): 246-255.

Ehnfors M. The development of the VIPS-model in Nordic countries. In: Oud N, ed. *ACENDIO 2002: Proceedings of the Special Conference of the Association of Common European Nursing Diagnoses, Interventions and Outcomes in Vienna.* Bern, Switzerland: Verlag Hans Huber; 2002.

Eisenberg JM. The effectiveness of clinical care: is there any evidence? Plenary paper presented at: ANA Council for Nursing Research Pre-conference on Research Utilization; June 1998; San Diego, Calif.

Elkan R, Blair M, Robinson JJA. Evidence-based practice and health visiting: the need for theoretical underpinnings for evaluation. *J Adv Nurs.* 2000;31(6):1316-1323.

Emden C, Young W. Theory development in nursing: Australian nurses advance global debate. *Aust J Adv Nurs.* 1987;4(3):22-40.

Eriksson K. Caring science in a new key. *Nurs Sci Q.* 2002;15:61-65.

Facione NC, Facione PA. Externalizing the critical thinking in knowledge development and clinical judgment. *Nurs Outlook.* 1996;44:129-136.

Fawcett J, Watson J, Neuman B, Walker PH, Fitzpatrick JJ. On nursing theories and evidence. *J Nurs Sch.* 2001;33(2):115-119.

Foster RL. Who is responsible for measuring nursing outcomes? *J Soc Pediatr Nurses.* 2001;6(3):107-108.

French P. What is the evidence on evidence-based nursing? an epistemological concern. *J Adv Nurs.* 2002;37(3):250-257.

Frey MA, Rooke L, Sieloff C, Messmer PR, Kameoka T. King's framework and theory in Japan, Sweden, and in the United States. *Image.* 1995;27:127-130.

Frisch N. What's in a name? *Nurs Diagn.* 1997;8(1):3-4.

Gamel C, Grypdonck M, Hengeveld M, Davis B. A method to develop a nursing intervention: the contribution of qualitative studies to the process. *J Adv Nurs.* 2001;33(6):806-819.

Good M, Moore SM. Clinical practice guidelines as a new source of middle-range theory: focus on acute pain. *Nurs Outlook.* 1996;44(2):74-79.

Goosen W. The international nursing minimum data set (J-NMDS): why do we need it? In: Oud N, ed. *ACENDIO 2002: Proceedings of the Special Conference of the Association of*

Common European Nursing Diagnoses, Interventions and Outcomes in Vienna. Bern, Switzerland: Verlag Hans Huber; 2002.

Graves J, Corcoran S. The study of nursing informatics. *Image.* 1989;21(4):227-231.

Greenwood J, Sullivan J, Spence K, McDonald M. Nursing scripts and the organizational infuences on critical thinking: report of a study of neonatal nurses' clinical reasoning. *J Adv Nurs.* 2000;31(5):1106-1114.

Gurrieri L. Unlocking a world of information. *Reflections Nurs Leadership.* 2000;26(4):8-9.

Hallett CE, Austin L, Caress A, Luker KA. Wound care in the community setting: clinical decision making in context. *J Adv Nurs.* 2000;31(4):783-793.

Hannah K, Ball M, Edwards M. *Introduction to Nursing Informatics.* New York, NY: Springer-Verlag; 1994.

Harding WT, Redmond RT, Corley MC, Nelson AS. Techniques in evaluating nursing expert systems: a case study. *Nurs Forum.* 1996;31(4):13-20.

Heller BR, Oros MT, Durney-Crowley J. The future of nursing education: 10 trends to watch. *Nurs Health Care Pers.* 2000;21(1): 9-13.

Hill-Westmoreland EE, Soeken K, Spellbring AM. A meta-analysis of fall prevention programs for the elderly. *Nurs Res.* 2002;51(1):1-8.

Hisama KK. International perspectives. The acceptance of nursing theory in Japan: a cultural perspective. *Nurs Sci Q.* 2001;14:255-259.

Holden RJ. In defence of Cartesian dualism and the hermeneutic horizon. *J Adv Nurs.* 1991;16:1375-1381.

Holmes CA. Resistance to positivist science in nursing: an assessment of the Australian literature. *Int J Nurs Pract.* 1996;2(4):172-181.

Im E, Meleis AI. A situation-specific theory of Korean immigrant women's menopausal transition. *Image.* 1999;31:333-338.

Iowa Intervention Project: a proposal to bring nursing into the information age. *Image.* 1997;29(3):275-281.

Ireson CL, Velotta CL. Accessibility to knowledge for research-based practice. In: Moorhead S, Delaney C, eds. *Information Systems Innovations for Nursing: New Visions and Ventures.* Thousand Oaks, Calif: Sage Publications; 1998: 94-105.

Jairath N, Fain, JA. A strategy for converting clinical data into research databases. *Nurs Res.* 1999;48(6):340-344.

Jennings BM. Evidence-based practice: the road best traveled? *Res Nurs Health.* 2000;23:343-345.

Jennings BM, Loan LA. Misconceptions among nurses about evidence-based practice. *J Nurs Schol.* 2001;33(2):121-127.

Jensen-Wunder L. Indian health initiatives: a nursing practice model. *Nurs Sci Q.* 2002;15:32-35.

Jonsdottir H. Nursing theories and their relation to knowledge development in Iceland. *Nurs Sci Q.* 2001;14:165-168.

Keenan GM, Stocker JR, Geo-Thomas AT, Soparkar NR, Barkauskas VH, Lee JL. The HANDS project: studying and refining the automated collection of cross-setting clinical data. *CIN: Computers, Informatics, Nursing.* 2002;20(3):89-100.

Kenney T. Nursing models fail in practice. *Br J Nurs.* 1993;2(2):133-136.

Ketefian S, Redman RW. Nursing science in the global community. *Image.* 1997;29:11-15.

Kimball B, O'Neil E. The evolution of a crisis: nursing in America. *Policies, Politics, & Nursing Practices.* 2001;2(3):180-186.

King I. *A Theory for Nursing: Systems, Concepts, Process.* New York, NY: Wiley; 1981.

Kirkevold M. Toward a practice theory of caring for patients with chronic skin disease. *Scholar Inquiry Nurs Pract.* 1993;7:37-57.

Kitson A. Using evidence to demonstrate the value of nursing. *Nurs Stand.* 1997;11(28):34-39.

Kolcaba K. Evolution of the midrange theory of comfort for outcomes research. *Nurs Outlook.* 2001;49(2):86-92.

Laschinger HKS, Sabiston, JA, Kutszcher L. Empowerment and staff nurse decision involvement in nursing work environments: testing Kanter's theory of structural power in organizations. *Res Nurs Health.* 1997;20:341-352.

Lauder W. The utility of self-care theory as a theoretical basis for self-neglect. *J Adv Nurs.* 2001;34:545-551.

Lauri S, Salanterä S, Chalmers C, Ekman S, Kim HS, Käppeli S, et al. An exploratory study of clinical decision-making in five countries. *J Nurs Sch.* 2001;33:83-90.

Lavin MA, Meyer G, Carlson J. A review of the use of nursing diagnosis in U.S. nurse practice acts. *Nurs Diagn.* 1999;10(2):57-64.

Lawler J. In search of an Australian identity. In: Gray G, Pratt R, eds. *Towards a Discipline of Nursing.* Melbourne, Australia: Churchill Livingstone; 1991.

Lee P. An analysis and evaluation of Casey's conceptual framework. *Int J Nurs Stud.* 1998;35(4):204-209.

Leininger MM. *Culture Care Diversity and Universality: A Theory of Nursing.* New York; NY: National League for Nursing; 1991.

Leino-Kilpi H, Suominen T. Nursing research in Finland from 1958 to 1995. *Image.* 1998;30:363-367.

Leveck ML, Jones CB. The nursing practice environment, staff retention, and quality of care. *Res Nurs Health.* 1996;19:331-343.

Liehr P, Smith MJ. Middle-range theory: spinning research and practice to create knowledge for the new millennium. *Adv Nurs Sci.* 1999;21(4):81-91.

Loxe J, Struthers R. A conceptual framework of nursing in Native American culture. *J Nurs Sch.* 2001;33:279-283.

Lundh U, Söder M, Waerness K. Nursing theories: a critical view. *Image.* 1988;20:36-40.

Lutzen K, da Silva AB. Delineating the domain of nursing science in Sweden—some relevant issues. *Vård i Norden.* 1995;15(1):4-7.

Maas ML, Johnson M, Moorhead S. Classifying nursing-sensitive patient outcomes. *Image.* 1996;28(4):295-301.

Major FA, Pepin JI, Légault AJ. Nursing knowledge in a mostly French-speaking Canadian province: from past to present. *Nurs Sci Q.* 2001;14:355-359.

Martin H, Rodrigues RJ, Delaney C, Nielsen GJ, Yan J, eds. *Building Standard-Based Nursing Information Systems.* Washington, DC: Pan American Health Organization; 2001.

Mason C. Guide to practice or load of rubbish? The influence of care plans on nursing practice in five clinical areas in northern Ireland. *J Adv Nurs.* 1999;29(2):380-387.

Mavundla TR, Poggenpoel M, Gmeiner A. A model of facilitative communication for the support of general hospital nurses nursing mentally ill people: part I: background, problem statement and research methodology. *Curationis.* 2001;24(1):7-14.

McConnell EA. Nursing publications outside the United States. *J Nurs Sch.* 2000;32:87-90.

McCormack B, Kitson A, Harvey G, Rycroft-Malone J, Titchen A, Seers, K. Getting evidence into practice: the meaning of context. *J Adv Nurs.* 2002;38(1):94-104.

Millenson MI. *Demanding medical evidence: doctors and accountability in the information age.* Chicago, Ill: University of Chicago Press; 1997.

Minshull J, Ross K, Turner J. The Human Needs Model of nursing. *J Adv Nurs.* 1986;11:643-649.

Mitchell PH, Ferketich S, Jennings BM. Quality health outcomes model. *Image.* 1998;30(1):43-46.

Moorhead S, Delaney C. Mapping nursing intervention data into the Nursing Intervention Classification (NIC): process and rules. *Nurs Diagn.* 1997;8(4):137-151.

Moorhead S, Delaney C., eds. *Information Systems Innovations for Nursing: New Visions and Ventures.* Thousand Oaks, Calif: Sage Publications; 1998.

Morales-Mann ET, Jiang SL. Applicability of Orem's conceptual framework: a cross-cultural point of view. *J Adv Nurs.* 1993;18:737-741.

Narayan SM, Corcoran-Perry S. Line of reasoning as a representation of nurses' clinical decision making. *Res Nurs Health.* 1997;20:353-364.

Needleman J, Buerhaus P, Mattke S, Stewart M, Zelevinsky K. Nurse staffing levels and the quality of care in hospitals. *New England Journal of Medicine.* 2002;346(22):1715-1722.

Nicoll LH. Tips, tools and techniques. Internet case management, Internet communication. *Lippincott's Case Management.* 2001;6(2):64-67.

Nightingale F. *Notes on hospitals.* London, England: Longman, Green, Longman, Roberts and Green; 1863: 175-176.

Nolan M, Lundh U, Tishelman C. Nursing's knowledge base: does it have to be unique? *Br J Nurs.* 1998;7(5):270, 272-276.

Norris JR. The Internet: extending our capacity for scholarly inquiry in nursing. *Nurs Sci Q.* 1999;12(3):197-201.

Orem D. *Nursing: Concepts of Practice.* 4th ed. St. Louis, Mo: Mosby; 1991.

Parse RR. *Hope: An International Human Becoming Perspective.* Sudbury, Mass: Jones & Bartlett; 1999.

Parse RR, ed. *Illuminations: The Human Becoming Theory in Practice and Research.* New York, NY: National League for Nursing; 1995.

Poggenpoel M. Psychiatric nursing research based on nursing for the whole person theory. *Curationis.* 1996;19(3):60-62.

Prowse MA, Lyne PA. Clinical effectiveness in the post-anaesthesia care unit: how nursing knowledge contributes to achieving intended patient outcomes. *J Adv Nurs.* 2000;31(5):1115-1124.

Radwin LE. Conceptualizations of decision making in nursing: analytic models and "knowing the patient." *Nurs Diagn.* 1995;6(1):16-22.

Reed J, Robbins I. Models of nursing: their relevance to the care of elderly people. *J Adv Nurs.* 1991;16:1350-1357.

Roberson MR, Kelley JH. Using Orem's theory in transcultural settings: a critique. *Nurs Forum.* 1996;31:22-28.

Roberts K. Evidence-based practice: an idea whose time has come. *Collegian.* 1998;5(3):24-27.

Rodgers SJ. The role of nursing theory in standards of practice: a Canadian perspective. *Nurs Sci Q.* 2000;13:260-262.

Roper N, Logan WW, Tierney AJ. *The Elements of Nursing.* 2nd ed. Edinburgh, Scotland: Churchill Livingstone; 1985.

Ruland CM, Moore SM. Theory construction based on standards of care: a proposed theory of the peaceful end of life. *Nurs Outlook.* 1998;46(4):169-175.

Sackett DL, Rosenberg WMC, Gray JAM, Haynes RB, Richardson WS. Evidence-based medicine: what it is and what it isn't. *British Medical Journal.* 1996;312(7023):71-72.

Sarvimäki A. Nursing care as a moral, practical, communicative and creative activity. *J Adv Nurs.* 1988;13:462-467.

Searle C. Nursing theories: what is our commitment? *Nurs RSA Verpleging.* 1988;3(2):15-17, 19, 21.

Shin KR. Developing perspectives on Korean nursing theory: the influences of Taoism. *Nurs Sci Q.* 2001;14:346-353.

Simon JM. Nursing diagnoses and outcomes. *Nurs Diagn.* 1998;9(2):47-48.

Sirra E. An approach to systematic nursing. *Nurs J India.* 1986;77(1):3-5, 28.

Smith CE, Pace K, Kochinda C, Kleinbeck SVM, Koehler J, Popkess-Vawter S. Caregiving effectiveness model evolution to a midrange theory of home care: a process for critique and replication. *Adv Nurs Sci.* 2002;25(1):50-64.

Smith L. Application of nursing models to a curriculum: some considerations. *Nurse Educ Today.* 1987;7(3):109-115.

Snyder M, Egan E, Nojima Y. Defining nursing interventions. *Image.* 1996;28(2):137-141.

Sparks SM, Rizzolo MA. World wide web search tools. *Image.* 1998;30(2):167-171.

Taylor JY. Womanism: a methodologic framework for African American women. *Adv Nurs Sci.* 1998;21(1):53-64.

Thomas L, Cullum N, McColl E. Clinical guidelines in nursing, midwifery and other professions allied to medicine. *Cochrane Review.* November 28, 1998.

Thomas L, McColl E, Cullum N. Effect of clinical guidelines in nursing midwifery, and the therapies: a systematic review of evaluations. *Quality in Health Care.* 1998;7:183-191.

Thompson C. A conceptual treadmill: the need for "middle ground" in clinical decision making theory in nursing. *J Adv Nurs.* 1999;30(5):1222-1229.

Tierney AJ. Nursing models: extant or extinct? *J Adv Nurs.* 1998;28:377-385.

Timmons S. The potential contribution of science to information technology implementation in health care. *CIN: Computers, Informatics, Nursing.* 2002;20(2):74-78.

Traynor M, Rafferty AM, Lewison G. Endogenous and exogenous research? Findings from a bibliometric study of UK nursing research. *J Adv Nurs.* 2001;34(2):212-222.

Turley JP. Toward a model for nursing informatics. *Image.* 1996;28(4):309-313.

Turton CLR. Ways of knowing about health: an Aboriginal perspective. *Adv Nurs Sci.* 1997;19(3):28-36.

Villarruel AM, Denyes MJ. Testing Orem's theory with Mexican Americans. *Image.* 1997;29:283-288.

Wake M, Coenan A. Nursing diagnosis in the International Classification for Nursing Practice (ICNP). *Nurs Diagn.* 1998;9(3):111-118.

Walker LO. Is integrative science necessary to improve nursing practice? *West J Nurs Res.* 1999;21(1):94-102.

Whall AL, Shin YH, Colling KB. A Nightingale-based model of dementia care and its relevance for Korean nursing. *Nurs Sci Q.* 1999;12:319-323.

Whitley GG. A critical time for nursing diagnosis research. *Nurs Diagn.* 1999;10(4):173-174.

Willman A. Nursing theory in education, practice, and research in Sweden. *Nurs Sci Q.* 2000;13:263-265.

Willman A, Stoltz P. Yes, no, or perhaps: reflections on Swedish human science nursing research development. *Nurs Sci Q.* 2002;15:66-70.

Wong FKY, Ho M, Chiu I, Lui WK, Chan C, Lee KM. Factors contributing to hospital readmission in a Hong Kong regional hospital: a case controlled study. *Nurs Res.* 2002;51(1):40-44.

Zielstorff RD, Tronni C, Basque J, Griffin JR, Welebob EM. Mapping nursing diagnosis nomenclatures for coordinated care. *Image.* 1998;30(4):369-373.

ADDITIONAL READINGS

Adams T. The idea of revolution in the development of nursing theory. *J Adv Nurs.* 1991;16:1487-1491.

Bailey J. Reflective practice: implementing theory. *Nurs Stand.* 1995;9(46):29-31.

Bakken-Henry S, Holzemer WL, Tallberg M, Grobe S, eds. *Informatics: The Infrastructure for Quality Assessment & Improvement in Nursing.* San Francisco, Calif: UC Nursing Press; 1994.

Barker PJ, Reynolds W, Stevenson C. The human science basis of psychiatric nursing: theory and practice. *J Adv Nurs.* 1997;25:660-667.

Bostrom I, Hall-Lord M, Larsson G, Wilde B. Nursing theory based changes of work organisation in an ICU: effects on quality of care. *Intensive Crit Care Nurs.* 1992;8(1):10-16.

Brieskorn-Zinke M. The relevance of health sciences for nursing [in German]. *Pflege.* 1998;11(3):129-134.

Castledine G. Where are the British models? Nursing models. *Nurs Times.* 1985;81(43):22.

Chalmers KI. Giving and receiving: an empirically derived theory on health visiting practice. *J Adv Nurs.* 1992;17:1317-1325.

Cook SH. Mind the theory/practice gap in nursing. *J Adv Nurs.* 1991;16:1462-1469.

Eldh A. Monograph review: critical appraisal: nursing theories in practice, education and research. *Theoria J Nurs Theory.* 2001;10(3):17-19.

Emden C. Nursing knowledge: an intriguing journey. *Aust J Adv Nurs.* 1987–1988;5(2):33-45.

Evans AM. Philosophy of nursing: future directions. *Aust Nz J Ment Health Nurs.* 1995;4(1):14-21.

Gould D. Teaching theories and models of nursing: implications for a common foundation programme for nurses. *Recent Adv Nurs.* 1989;(24):93-105.

Gray G, Pratt R. *Scholarship in the Discipline of Nursing.* Melbourne, Australia: Churchill Livingstone; 1995.

Gray G, Pratt R. *Towards a Discipline of Nursing.* Melbourne, Australia: Churchill Livingstone; 1991.

Greenwood J. Reflective practice: a critique of the work of Argyris and Schon. *J Adv Nurs.* 1993;18:1183-1187.

Grobe SJ. The infrastructure for quality assessment and quality improvement. In: Bakken-Henry S, Holzemer WL, Tallberg M, Grobe S, eds. *Informatics: The Infrastructure for Quality Assessment & Improvement in Nursing.* San Francisco, Calif: UC Nursing Press; 1994.

Grobe SJ, Pluyter-Wenting ESP, eds. *Nursing Informatics: An International Overview for Nursing in a Technological Era.* Amsterdam, Netherlands: Elsevier; 1994.

Hauge S. From focusing on illness to focusing on health in nursing [in Norwegian]. *Vård i Norden.* 1997;17(1):18-24.

Hopkins S, McSherry R. Debate: is there a great divide between nursing theory and practice? *Nurs Times.* 2000;96(17):16.

Kyriacos U, van der Walt A. Attitudes of diploma-prepared and graduate registered nurses towards nursing models: a comparative study. *Curationis.* 1996;19(3):2-6.

Laschinger HK, Duff V. Attitudes of practicing nurses towards theory-based nursing practice. *Can J Nurs Adm.* 1991;4(1):6-10.

Lewis T. Leaping the chasm between nursing theory and practice. *J Adv Nurs.* 1988;13:345-351.

Mattice M. Parse's theory of nursing in practice: a manager's perspective. *Can J Nurs Adm.* 1991;4(1):11-13.

Meleis AI. Theoretical nursing: today's challenges, tomorrow's bridges. *Nurs Pap.* 1987;19(1):45-56.

Mulholland J. Assimilating sociology: critical reflections on the "sociology in nursing" debate. *J Adv Nurs.* 1997;25:844-852.

Muller E, Reipschlager C. The drawing up of a classification system for nursing science for the University Library in Bremen—a contribution to the development of nursing as a science [in German]. *Pflege.* 1997;10(5):292-298.

Norberg A, Wickstrom E. The perception of Swedish nurses and nurse teachers of the integration of theory with nursing practice. An explorative qualitative study. *Nurse Educ Today.* 1990;10(1):38-43.

Oud N, ed. *ACENDIO 2002: Proceedings of the Special Conference of the Association of Common European Nursing Diagnoses, Interventions and Outcomes in Vienna.* Bern, Switzerland Verlag Hans Huber; 2002.

Quiquero A, Knights D, Meo CO. Theory as a guide to practice: staff nurses choose Parse's theory. *Can J Nurs Adm.* 1991;4(1):14-16.

Scott H. More clinical skills but not at the expense of theory. *Br J Nurs.* 1999;8:910.

Smith JP. *Models, Theories, and Concepts.* London, England: Blackwell Scientific; 1994.

Smith M, Cusack L. The Ottawa Charter—from nursing theory to practice: insights from the area of alcohol and other drugs. *Int J Nurs Pract.* 2000;6(4):168-173.

Story EL, Ross MM. Family centered community health nursing and the Betty Neuman Systems Model. *Nurs Pap.* 1986;18(2):77-88.

Tornstam L. Caring for the elderly: introducing the theory of gerotranscendence as a supplementary frame of reference for caring for the elderly. *Scand J Caring Sci.* 1996;10(3):144-150.

Wang Y, Li X. Cross-cultural nursing theory and Chinese nursing today [in Chinese]. *Chinese Nurs Res.* 2000;14(6):231-232.

Warren J, Hoskins L. NANDA's nursing diagnosis taxonomy: a nursing database. In: *ANA Steering Committee on Databases to Support Clinical Nursing Practice.* Washington, DC: ANA Publishing; 1995.

Zielstorff, RD, Hudgings CI, Grobe SJ, and the National Commission on Nursing Implementation Project Task Force on Nursing Information Systems. *Next-Generation Nursing Information Systems.* Washington, DC: ANA Publishing; 1993.

Index

Page numbers in *italics* denote figures; those followed by "t" denote tables.